Drugs of Abuse
Gastroenterology: Problems in Primary Care
Medical Care of the Adolescent Athlete
Medical Procedures for Referral
Neurology: Problems in Primary Care
Orthopaedics: Problems in Primary Care
Patient Care Emergency Handbook
Patient Care Flowchart Manual
Patient Care Procedures for Your Practice
Pulmonary Medicine: Problems in Primary Care
Questions & Answers on AIDS
Sexually Transmitted Diseases
Urology: Problems in Primary Care

PRACTICE MANAGEMENT

365 Ways to Manage the Business Called Private Practice
Achieving Profitability with a Medical Office System
Choosing and Using a Medical Office Computer
Computerizing Your Medical Office
Designing and Building Your Professional Office
Doctor Business
Encyclopedia of Practice and Financial Management
Getting Paid for What You Do
Health Information Management
Managing Medical Office Personnel
Managing the Physician's Office Laboratory
Marketing Strategies for Physicians
Medical Marketing Handbook
Medical Practice Handbook
Medical Software, Systems & Services Directory
Medical Staff Privileges
Negotiating Managed Care Contracts
New Practice Handbook
Patient Satisfaction
Patients Build Your Practice
Physician's Office Laboratory
Professional and Practice Development
Promoting Your Medical Practice
Starting in Medical Practice
Spanish/English Handbook for Medical Professionals

**AVAILABLE FROM YOUR LOCAL MEDICAL
BOOK STORE OR CALL 1-800-MED-SHOP**

OTHER PMIC TITLES OF INTEREST

CODING AND REIMBURSEMENT

Codelink®
CPT Coders Choice®, Thumb Indexed
CPT TimeSaver®, Ring Binder, Tab Indexed
CPT & HCPCS Coding Made Easy!
HCPCS Coders Choice®
Health Insurance Carrier Directory
ICD-9-CM, Coders Choice®, Thumb Indexed
ICD-9-CM, TimeSaver®, Ring Binder, Tab Indexed
ICD-9-CM Coding For Physicians Offices
ICD-9-CM Coding Made Easy!
Medicare Rules & Regulations
Physician Fees Guide
Reimbursement Manual for the Medical Office
Working with Insurance and Managed Care Plans

FINANCIAL MANAGEMENT

Accounts Receivable Management for the Medical Practice
Business Ventures for Physicians
Financial Planning Workbook for Physicians
Financial Valuation of Your Practice
Pension Plan Strategies
Physician Financial Planning in a Changing Environment
Securing Your Assets
Selling or Buying a Medical Practice

RISK MANAGEMENT

Law, Liability and Ethics for Medical Office Personnel
Malpractice Depositions
Malpractice: Managing Your Defense
Medical Risk Management
Testifying in Court

DICTIONARIES AND OTHER REFERENCE

Drug Interactions Index
Isler's Pocket Dictionary
Medical Acronyms, Eponyms and Abbreviations
Medical Phrase Index
Medical Word Building
Medico-Legal Glossary

**AVAILABLE FROM YOUR LOCAL MEDICAL
BOOK STORE OR CALL 1-800-MED-SHOP**

MEDICO MNEMONICA

A Collection of
Fun, Ribald,
Irreverent and
Quite Witty
Mnemonics for
Medical Students

E.S. Marlowe, M.D.

Library of Congress Cataloging-in-Publication Data

Marlowe, E.S. (Evan S.), 1969-
    Medico menomica : medical school mnemonics / written
and compiled by E.S. Marlowe.
      p. cm.
    ISBN 1-57066-056-5 (pbk. : alk. paper)
    1. Medical sciences--Examinations, questions, etc.
2. Mnemonics.
I. Title.
    [DNLM: 1.   Medicine--examination   questions.
2. Association Learning.   W 18.2 M349m 1997]
R834.5.M37 1997
610'.76--dc21
DNLM/DLC
for Library of Congress   96-49033
                                              CIP

Practice Management Information Corporation
4727 Wilshire Boulevard, Suite 300
Los Angeles, California 90010
1-800-MED-SHOP
e-mail: MEDICALBOOKSTORE.COM

Printed in the United States of America

ABOUT THE AUTHOR

Evan S. Marlowe, M.D., compiled *Medico Mnemonica* while in medical school studying for his boards. He graduated from the University of Arkansas for Medical Sciences, in Little Rock. Originally from Southern California, he next spent a "brutal year" of surgery training in Portland, Oregon. Young Dr. Marlowe says he thought medical school was hell, but after this year, realized it was merely purgatory. He subsequently pursued a career in physiatry.

DISCLAIMER

The information presented in this book is based on the experience and interpretations of the author. Though all of the information has been carefully researched and checked for accuracy and completeness, neither the author nor the publisher accept any responsibility or liability with regard to errors, omissions, misuse or misinterpretation.

CONTENTS

PREFACE

Although it is generally accepted that the first two years of medical school are designed to prepare the student for what is to come, few in the Establishment will openly admit that these years are also a glorified fraternity hazing party. In the typical school, you start off with gross anatomy, a gruesome affair that costs you your better-smelling friends. In neuroanatomy you discover parts of the body you probably won't run across again during your practice (and if you do, you know you've gone too far).

While taking physiology and biochemistry, you are expected to know what each molecule in the human body is intended for, and in pathology you learn what it isn't intended for. Behavioral science tells you how each molecule affects patient compliance and what each molecule will cost the health care system. In addition, the medical student must learn about every micro-organism known to science (and, of course, how to culture them all, just in case the lab techs all go on strike for a week), as well as every drug used medicinally or in research.

Most everything I remember from my first two years of medical school is associated with a mnemonic. I am convinced I could not have made it otherwise; there's just too much to learn in too short of a time to try to actually "get to know" each iota of knowledge. The contents of this book, despite its pretentious title, are intended to lighten your load a bit. Needless to say, many things you'll come across *must* be memorized, and no mnemonic can help you there.

In writing and compiling this book, I tried to avoid the "Some Say Marry Money" types of mnemonics (see page 3), since these are usually too difficult to recall. Most of the time, the solution can be found by dissecting and reinterpreting the given item. For example, a question frequently asked is, "What toxin is dimercaprol used for... organic or inorganic mercury?" Well, even if the question hadn't told you that it treated mercury poisoning, you could have weeded it out of the word (di**MERC**aprol). And the answer is also given in the word; you treat **I**norganic mercury (d**I**mercaprol) and never organic mercury poisoning. I find these types of mnemonics far easier and more useful, so I've strived to stress these.

Another favorite method of mine is to think up a word like SALT, so when you are asked to recall what cell in the testes makes testosterone, you'll think: **S**ertolis make **ABP** while **L**eydigs make **T**estosterone. Of course, the drawback to these is you may start to confuse SALT with CONE or BANG. To avoid mixing up the mnemonics, I recommend writing each one down in your notes when you are introduced to the topic during your medical school course. Temporal spacing of this nature reduces the confusion. Finally, although I've taken extra precautions to assure accuracy, always trust your instructors or textbooks when in doubt of something.

Many schools give students about a month to prepare for the boards, which is really not enough time compared to the summer one has to study for the MCAT. I was warned beforehand not to spend too much time on anatomy, and this was good advice. If your board exam is like mine and those that preceded me, you should spend most your time on pathology, physiology and microbiology.

And most importantly, always keep your sanity...

Evan S. Marlowe, M.D.,
Summer, 1997

GROSS ANATOMY

How is the spinal cord arranged?

SAME DAVE

Sensory is **A**fferent   **D**orsal has **A**fferent roots
Motor is **E**fferent   **V**entral has **E**fferent roots

Sympathetic innervation is associated with an excited state, like "Sympathy for the Devil" by the Stones. *Parasympathetic* is just the opposite.

How does the brachial plexus divide?

Robert	**R**oots
Taylor	**T**runks
Drinks	**D**ivisions
Cold	**C**ords
Beer	**B**ranches

What is the innervation to the diaphragm?
C3, 4, and 5 keep you alive.

What is the innervation to the penis?
S2, 3, and 4 keep the penis off the floor.

How does the autonomic nervous system control the penis?
Point and **S**hoot:
Parasympathetics cause erection (point) and
    urination (pee);
Sympathetics cause ejaculation (shoot)

Many neurovascular bundles in the body can be remembered as VAN (**v**ein - **ar**tery - **n**erve). Here is a table of important VANs:

The clavipectoral fascia is pierced by...	Cephalic (V) Thoracoacromial (A) LATERAL pectoral (N)
The inguinal region contains... *(medial to lateral)*	Empty space (lymph duct) Femoral (V) Femoral (A) Femoral (N) <div align="right">(it spells my name: EVAN)</div>
The parotid gland contains...	Retromandibular (V) External carotid branches (A) Facial (N)
The carotid sheath/triangle contains...	Internal jugular (V) Common and internal carotid (A) Vagus (N)
The cubital fossa contains a variant (TAN)... *(lateral to medial)*	Biceps TENDON Brachial (A) Median (N)
The popliteal fossa contains...	Popliteal (V) Popliteal (A) Tibial (N)

The intercostal spaces also each contain an intercostal vein, artery, and nerve.

What are the cranial nerves?
Several mnemonics exist, so take your choice (unfortunately, I can not claim responsibility for these):

I.	OLFACTORY	Oh!	On
II.	OPTIC	Oh!!	Old
III.	OCULOMOTOR	Oh!!!	Olympus'
IV.	TROCHLEAR	To	Towering
V.	TRIGEMINAL	Touch	Tops
VI.	ABDUCENS	And	A
VII.	FACIAL	Feel	Finn
VIII.	VESTIBULOCOCHLEAR	Veronica's	And (for Auditory)
IX.	GLOSSOPHARYNGEAL	Gaping	German
X.	VAGUS	Vagina	Viewed
XI.	ACCESSORY	And	Some (for Spinal)
XII.	HYPOGLOSSAL	Hymen	Hopps

Which cranial nerves are motor, sensory, or both?

I.	SENSORY	Some	Some
II.	SENSORY	Say	Say
III.	MOTOR	Marry	Marry
IV.	MOTOR	Money	Money
V.	BOTH	But	But
VI.	MOTOR	My	My
VII.	BOTH	Boyfriend	Boyfriend
VIII.	SENSORY	Says	Says
IX.	BOTH	Better	Bigger
X.	BOTH	Brains	Breasts
XI.	MOTOR	Make	Matter
XII.	MOTOR	Millions	More

Whichever mnemonic you choose, do not replace "boyfriend" with "brother," or you might start thinking "sister" and conclude the facial nerve only contains sensory fibers.

Name the important holes in the base of the skull from the internal perspective (from anterior to posterior):

Cleaning	foramen **C**ecum
Clinton's	**C**ribiform foramina
SOFt	**S**uperior **O**rbital **F**issure
Rubbers	foramen **R**otundum
Out	foramen **O**vale
She	foramen **S**pinosum
Lamented,	foramen **L**acerum
"I A M	**I**nternal **A**uditory **M**eatus
Just	**J**ugular foramen
His	**H**ypoglossal canal
Maid!"	foramen **M**agnum

The optic canal lies adjacent to the SOF.

What cranial nerves exit the jugular foramen?

> 9, 10, 11
> Jugular foramen

(Keep reciting this one until it sticks...)

What passes through the cavernous sinus?

> The Cavernous Sinus...
> Where no MAN has gone before!

The internal carotid A. and cranial nerves 3 through 6, except the MANdibular branch of 5 (V_3).

Through what bones do cranial nerves 1 through 12 exit the skull?

TOES (**T**emporal, **O**ccipital, **E**thmoid, **S**phenoid):

T	O	E	S
7 8 9 10 11	12 1	2 3 4 5 6

Here is what the nasal conchae receive:

SUPERIOR MEATUS posterior ethmoidal air cells sphenoidal sinus
MIDDLE MEATUS everything else
INFERIOR MEATUS nasolacrimal duct

What is adduction?

When you ADDuct, you are ADDing a part of the body towards the midline. Abduction moves it away from the midline.

What are the branches of the mandibular sensory (V_3) nerve?

BAM!

Buccal
Auriculotemporal
Mental

(These nerves let you feel when you have been socked in the jaw.)

What innervates the extrinsic eye muscles?
The classic mnemonic is **LR$_6$SO$_4$**:

- **L**ateral **R**ectus gets CN **6**, **S**uperior **O**blique gets CN **4**.
- All other muscles receive CN 3 (oculo-motor nerve).

This mnemonic may be sufficient for you, but I rely on the following:

- Cranial nerve FOUR (trochlear) lets you look at your FOREarm (*down* and out), via the superior oblique. This is in contrast to the *inferior* oblique which lets you look *up* and out.
- *Lateral* rectus lets you turn your eye out *laterally* (i.e., abduct it), so the muscle receives the abducens nerve (CN 6).
- All other muscles receive CN 3 and do what their names imply.

What is the innervation of the two digastrics?
Heinz 57:

> Anterior digastric is cranial nerve 5
> Posterior digastric is cranial nerve 7

(Front to back, the way you'd eat a hamburger.)

Where do you find elastic cartilage?
Elastic cartilage lets you talk and listen, so you find it in the external ear, the auditory tube, and parts of the larynx.

What are the branches of the facial nerve within the parotid gland?

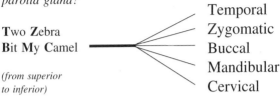

Two **Z**ebra
Bit **M**y **C**amel

*(from superior
to inferior)*

Temporal
Zygomatic
Buccal
Mandibular
Cervical

Where do you find the brachial plexus and phrenic nerve in relation to the scalenes?
The **B**rachial plexus runs **B**ehind the anterior scalene muscle. The **PHR**enic nerve runs in **FR**ont of the muscle.

What are the layers of the scalp?

SCALP

Skin
Connective tissue
Aponeurosis
Loose **A**reolar tissue
Periosteum

- The ESOPHAGUS is the most muscular part of the GI (gastrointestinal tract).
- All GI sections have inner circular and outer longitudinal muscles except the PHARYNX, which is backwards.

Which pterygoid muscle opens the mouth and moves it forward?
The LATERAL pterygoid.
Just think of the two pterygoids as barn doors: associate **lateral** with **open** and **medial** with **shut**.

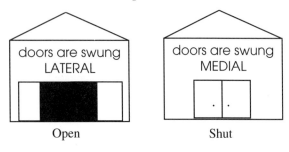

Open   Shut

How is the larynx organized?

- ONLY THE POSTERIOR CRICOARYTENOIDS ABDUCT.
- The nerve supply to the muscles is the recurrent laryngeal nerve *except* the CRICOTHYROID which gets the external laryngeal nerve.
- The mucosa is innervated above the true folds by the INTERNAL LARYNGEAL nerve.
- The mucosa is innervated below the true folds by the RECURRENT LARYNGEAL nerve.
- Blood to the area above the true folds comes from the SUPERIOR LARYNGEAL artery.
- Blood to the area below the true folds comes from the INFERIOR LARYNGEAL artery.

In what order do the inferior vena cava, aorta and esophagus pass through the diaphragm?
Dorsal to ventral, it's alphabetical (A E I):

Remember, the aorta must be protected at all costs, so it's placed between the spine and all of the other organs.

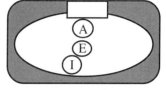

ventral

Arrange the cricoid, hyoid, and thyroid cartilage from superior to inferior:

Hate This Class

> **H**yoid bone
> **T**hyroid cartilage
> **C**ricoid cartilage

What are the muscles of the deep back?
They compose a **SET** of muscles:

> **S**plenius
> **E**rector spinae
> **T**ransversospinalis

How are the muscles of the erector spinae arranged?
They **SLI**de down the spine and out *(medial to lateral)*:

> **S**pinalis
> **L**ongissimus
> **I**liocostalis

The jugular veins have symmetrical distributions, such that the external and internal branches drain separately into the subclavians on both sides. The arteries, however, are not symmetrical:

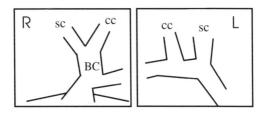

On the LEFT side, the common carotid (cc) and subclavian (sc) both come STRAIGHT off the aortic arch. On the right side, they don't (they branch from the brachiocephalic trunk [BC]).

This one can be remembered utilizing the old stereotype that if a man wears an earring in his right ear, he is gay, and if he wears it in his LEFT ear, he is STRAIGHT.

What are the branches of the external carotid artery?

Superior thyroid	**S**ome
Ascending pharyngeal	**A**ncient
Lingual	**L**overs
Facial	**F**ind
Occipital	**O**ld
Posterior auricular	**P**ositions
Maxillary	**M**ore
Superficial temporal	**S**atisfying

What are the branches of the maxillary artery?

DAMn I'M PISseD!

(From back to front, roughly.)

Deep auricular (**D**)
Anterior tympanic (**A**)
Middle meningeal (**M**)
Inferior alveolar (**I**$_A$)
Mastication muscles (**M**)
Posterior superior
  alveolar (**P**)
Infraorbital (**I**)
Sphenopalatine (**S**)
Descending palatine (**D**)

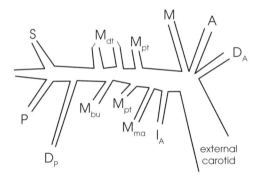

Note that the muscles of mastication receive:

- Buccal (M$_{bu}$)
- Masseteric (M$_{ma}$)
- Deep Temporals (M$_{dt}$)
- Pterygoids (M$_{pt}$)

What are the rotator cuff muscles?
SITS:

> **Supraspinatus**
> **Infraspinatus**
> **Teres minor**
> **Subscapularis**

These three are LATERAL rotators, while subscapularis is a medial rotator

The supraspinatus, infraspinatus, and teres minor also form THE GREAT SIT, since they all insert into the GREATer tubercle of the humerus.

The subscapularis is most like what other muscle in innervation, arterial supply, and action?

The teres MAJOR.

If you understand that the teres major is believed to be a derivative of the subscapularis that has migrated dorsally, you should remember everything about it.

What nerves provide sensation to the arm?

Lateral: **ARM**
  Axillary nerve
  Radial nerve
  Musculocutaneous nerve

Posterior: Radial nerve
Medial: Medial cord *(via medial brachial & antebrachial nerves)*

How are the respiratory muscles interior to the ribcage arranged?
TAPS:

Anterior

Transversus are along the **A**nterior body wall.

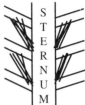

*T*RANSVERSUS muscles

Posterior

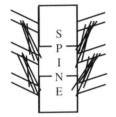

Subcostals are along the **P**osterior body wall.

*S*UBCOSTAL muscles

Here are some important dermatomes:
For the hand, make the Mr. Spock gesture ("live long and prosper"). The thumb gets T6, the second and third fingers get T7, and the last two fingers get T8.

> The nipple is T4
> The umbilicus is T10

What nerves innervate the fingertips?
Make the money gesture by rubbing your thumb across your lateral three digits. When you do this, the tips of the thumb, index, and middle fingers are in

contact. Notice only the lateral half of the ring finger is involved. Hence, M is for Money and MEDIAN nerve. The tip of the pinky and the medial half of the ring finger receive the ulnar nerve.

What are the superficial extensors of the forearm?
(lateral to medial)

CuRLy's on the	**CRL** is **C**arpi **R**adialis **L**ongus
CuRB	**CRB** is **C**arpi **R**adialis **B**revis
DIGging	**DIG** is **DIG**itorum
a DuMb	**DM** is **D**igiti **M**inimi
CARPooL	**CARPUL** is **CARP**i **UL**naris

- The three pollicis muscles lie deep to these, as does extensor indicis.
- The extensor compartment receives the posterior interosseous nerve, except CRL which gets the radial nerve directly.

> The brachioradialis divides these two compartments on the lateral side.

What are the superficial flexors of the forearm?
(lateral to medial)

	CR is **C**arpi **R**adialis
The CaRPooL	**PL** is **P**almaris **L**ongus
FLooDS	**FLDS** is **FL**exor **D**igitorum **S**uperficialis
so FuCk yoU	**FCU** is **F**lexor **C**arpi **U**lnaris

Deep to these are *F. digitorum profundus* and *F. pollicus longus*.

Where do most of the flexors originate?
They begin MEDIALLY and move distally.
Remember this by grasping the distal end of your right humerus with the fingers of your left hand covering the cubital fossa.

The flexor compartment receives the median nerve with two exceptions:
1. FCU which says, "Fuck you, I want my own nerve!" and steals the ulnar nerve.
2. Flexor Digitorum Profundus, which has dual innervation...

The nerves to the flexor digitorum profundus can be remembered as follows:

> YOU AND ME
> DIG THE PROFESSOR (well, not *really* me...)

In other words, U (ulnar) and ME (median) DIG the PROF (digitorum profundus), but not *really* me, since a branch off the median nerve called the anterior interosseus innervates it.

How do the interosseous muscles of the hand operate?
PAD and **DAB**

> **P**almers **AD**duct
> **D**orsals **AB**duct

(Remember that the hand is supine in anatomical position.)

What is supine?
When your hands are holding a bowl of soup, they are supine.

How are the carpal bones arranged?

Some **L**overs **T**ry **P**ositions
That **T**hey **C**an't **H**andle

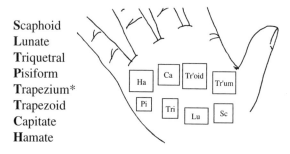

Scaphoid
Lunate
Triquetral
Pisiform
Trapezium*
Trapezoid
Capitate
Hamate

*(*the trapezi**UM** is near the th**UM**b)*

What are the muscles of the thenar eminence?
ABBY and OPPY are Friends.
The **AB**ductor (*not* adductor) pollicis brevis, **OP**ponens pollicis, and the **F**lexor pollicis brevis comprise the thenar eminence.

Which component of the neurovascular bundle transmitted by the inguinal canal is not within the femoral sheath?
The Nerve is Not:

What does the recurrent median nerve innervate?

LEFTOVER MEATLOAF

Leftover is **RECURRENT**
Meat is **MED**ian nerve
LOAF is:

Lateral lumbricals

Opponens pollicus
Abductor pollicus brevis
Flexor pollicus brevis
} *these three are thenar muscles*

What nerve and artery run over the surface of the serratus anterior?
The long thoracic nerve can be cut during mastectomy and cause wing scapula.
Don't confuse this nerve with its accompanying artery...

Lo**N**g thoracic **N**erve
LAteral thoracic **A**rtery

The **IN**direct hernia goes **IN** the scrotum or hernia sac (while the direct is outside) and the inferior epigastric artery is palpated **IN**terior (i.e., medial) to the herniation.

What are the structures running along the anterior body wall, viewed from within?

IOU:

   Inferior epigastric A and V

   Obliterated umbilical A

   Urachus

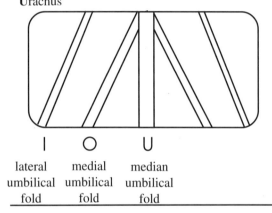

I	O	U
lateral umbilical fold	medial umbilical fold	median umbilical fold

What structures pass behind the medial malleolus of the ankle? (anterior to posterior)

Tom, Dick, ANd Harry:

   Tom is **TIBIALIS** posterior tendon

   Dick is flexor **DIGITORUM** longus tendon

   ANd is posterior tibial **ARTERY** and tibial **NERVE**

   Harry is flexor **HALLUCIS** longus

GROSS ANATOMY QUIZ

1. Which does not contain a vein-artery-nerve group?
   a. The parotid gland
   b. The cubital fossa
   c. The popliteal fossa
   d. The carotid sheath

2. Which is incorrect?
   a. T3, 4, and 5 innervate the diaphragm.
   b. Parasympathetics cause penile erection.
   c. S2, 3 and 4 innervate the penis.
   d. Sympathetics aid in the "fight or flight" response.

3. Which is matched correctly?
   a. CN I ... optic nerve
   b. CN V... trochlear nerve
   c. CN X ... vestibulocochlear
   d. CN XI ... accessory

4. Which hole in the floor of the skull is closest to the foramen magnum?
   a. Internal auditory meatus
   b. Hypoglossal canal
   c. Foramen cecum
   d. Foramen lacerum

5. Through which hole does CN 10 leave the skull?
   a. F. spinosum
   b. F. cecum
   c. Jugular foramen
   d. F. lacerum

6. Through what bone does the hypoglossal nerve exit the skull?
   a. Ethmoid
   b. Occipital
   c. Sphenoid
   d. Temporal

7. Which does not empty into the middle meatus of the nose?
   a. Maxillary sinus
   b. Frontonasal duct
   c. Nasolacrimal duct
   d. Ethmoidal air cells

8. Which is not a branch of CN V_3?
   a. Zygomatic
   b. Buccal
   c. Mental
   d. Auriculotemporal

9. What opens the jaw?
   a. Temporalis
   b. Medial pterygoids
   c. Buccal
   d. Lateral pterygoids

For questions 10-12, label the following structures as they pass through the diaphragm:

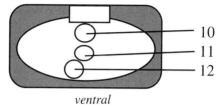

ventral

    a. Superior vena cava
    b. Inferior vena cava
    c. Esophagus
    d. Lungs
    e. Aorta

13. What is the order of structures from superior to inferior?
    a. Hyoid - Cricoid - Thyroid
    b. Thyroid - Cricoid - Hyoid
    c. Hyoid - Thyroid - Cricoid
    d. Cricoid - Hyoid - Thyroid

14. Which is a branch of the external carotid artery?
    a. Deep auricular
    b. Infraorbital
    c. Masseteric
    d. Facial

15. Which is a branch of the maxillary artery?
    a. Middle meningeal
    b. Lingual
    c. Occipital
    d. Superior thyroid

16. What innervates the area of skin covering the section of deltoid that abducts the arm?
    a. Musculocutaneous
    b. Medial brachial
    c. Axillary
    d. Radial

17. What dermatome covers the umbilicus?
    a. T6
    b. T8
    c. T10
    d. T12

From the following list, choose the one correct answer for questions 18-20:
    a. T5 and ulnar nerve
    b. T5 and median nerve
    c. T6 and ulnar
    d. T6 and median
    e. T7 and ulnar
    f. T7 and median
    g. T8 and ulnar
    h. T8 and median

18. What innervates the fifth digit (pinky) fingertip?

19. What innervates the thumb fingertip?

20. What innervates the middle digit fingertip?

21. A nerve is severed in the arm, but the flexor digitorum profundus is unaffected. The nerve severed is most likely:
    a. The median nerve
    b. The anterior interosseous nerve
    c. The ulnar nerve
    d. The radial nerve

22. Which is not innervated by the recurrent median nerve?
    a. Adductor pollicus brevis
    b. Opponens pollicus
    c. Abductor pollicus brevis
    d. Lateral lumbricals

23. What structure runs within the median umbilical fold?
    a. Inferior epigastric artery
    b. Median umbilical artery
    c. Urachus
    d. Obliterated umbilical artery

24. An inguinal herniation that enters the scrotum is commonly referred to as:
    a. Indirect
    b. Direct
    c. Groinal
    d. Intraorchal

25. What runs behind the medial malleolus?
    a. Flexor pollicus longus tendon
    b. Tibialis anterior tendon
    c. Flexor hallucis longus tendon
    d. Extensor digitorum longus tendon

MICROANATOMY AND EMBRYOLOGY

What are the parts of a microscope?

SCOPE

Source
Condenser lens
Objective lens
Projective lens
Eyepiece

What are the extraneuronal cells of the PNS?
These begin with **S**:
Schwann cells and **S**atellite cells. The CNS cells don't begin with S.

What are the layers of the skin?
Ed's pal's ready.

ED is **E**pi**D**ermis
PAL is **PA**pi**L**lary layer of dermis
Ready is **RETI**, the **RETI**cular layer

Where are Hassall bodies?
The THYMUS is too much of a hassle (Hassall), so it involutes early in life.

How many days does the RBC typically survive?

RBC lives **123**

Approximately 123 days.

Where are collagens I and II found?
Type **ONE** is in b**ONE**, type two is in cartilage.

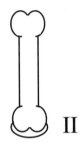

What is the A band of muscle?
The D**A**RK part of the sarcomere is the **A** band.
The L**I**GHT part is the **I** band.

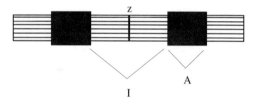

Which cells of the pars distalis are acidophilic?
MenS**es** (which, like acidophilic cells, is red).
M = **M**ammatroph-releasing cells (PRL)
S = **S**omatotroph-releasing cells (GH)

Most other cells are basophilic. If this seems too hard to recall, try...
   SoMa (as in cell body) = **So**mato / **Ma**mmatroph

What do chief cells release?
The two P's...

> **P**epsin (in the stomach)
> **PTH** (in the parathyroid gland)

What are the stages of mitosis?
IPMAT

> Interphase, Prophase, Metaphase,
> Anaphase, Telophase

What stages do the ova get stuck in?

> **PROPHASE I** → **METAPHASE II**
> until ovulation   until fertilization

What are the important infectious teratogens?
ToRCHeS

To is **To**xoplasma gondii	*brain calcifications scattered*
R is **R**ubella	*rubella triad*
C is **C**MV	*calcifications CircuMVent ventricles*
He is **He**rpes	*rarely transplacental; usually at birth*
S is **S**yphilis	*Hutchinson's triad*

What cells make testosterone in the testes?

Aside from the adrenal cortex, the interstitial Leydig cells make testosterone. The Sertoli cells wrap around the dividing sperm and produce androgen-binding protein (ABP) and inhibin. Use the following mnemonic to remember this:

SALT

Sertolis make ABP, while Leydigs make Testosterone

SILT also tells you the Sertoli cells make Inhibin.

What is capacitation?

When it greets the ovum, the sperm takes off its **CAP** (in the **CAP**acitation reaction). In other words, the sperm removes its **HAT**, releasing...

Hyaluronidase
Acrosin
Trypsin-like enzymes

When does organogenesis occur?

The preorganogenesis period encompasses the first two weeks. After that, organs begin to develop roughly in the following order (**CELTS**):

week 3	**C**NS and **C**ardiac (heart)
week 4	**E**yes, **E**ars, **E**xtremities
week 5	**L**ips
week 6	**T**eeth, **T**op of mouth (palate)
week 7	**S**ex

The head (anterior neuropore) closes before the tail (posterior neuropore), and the arms form before the legs.

> **HEAD** before **TAIL**
> **ARMS** before **LEGS**

How do the testes and bladder "migrate" during development?

> The bladder goes **UP**
> The testes go **DOWN**

What are the pharyngeal arch derivatives?

ARCH 1:	**M**asticators and **M**ylohyoid **T**ensors veli palatini and **T**ympani **V** (5th cranial nerve)	**MTV** (anterior digastric as well; see p. 6)
ARCH 2:	**VII** (7th cranial nerve) **ST**ylohyoid and **ST**apedius	**7th St.** (street) (posterior digastric as well, see p. 6)
ARCH 3:	**IX** (9th cranial nerve) Stylopharyngeus	
ARCH 4:	**X** (10th cranial nerve) everything else	

Notice the nerves in order are 5, 7, 9, 10; these are also the factors inhibited in vitamin K deficiency (if you haven't learned this part of pathology, this won't help you). Also note that nerves in each arch innervate the accompanying structures.

What does the tetralogy of Fallot consist of?
When you **SHOVE** a person from a window, they **FALL OuT**.

SHOVE	**S**tenosis of the pulmonary artery **H**ypertrophy of the right ventricle **O**verriding aorta **V**entricular septal defect **E**rythropoiesis stimulated

(This mnemonic appears courtesy of Dr. Robert Burns.)

What are the right-to-left heart shunts?

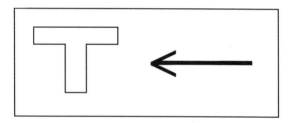

Above is a diagram to help remember that we are pointing left. Color the T in blue. Point left to the blue T. Right-to-left shunts are associated with the following:
1) Cyanosis (hence blue)
2) Defects starting with T:
   • Tetralogy of Fallot
   • Tricuspid atresia
   • Transposition of the great vessels
   • Truncus arteriosus

What are the GI autonomic plexuses?

> MeissNER's is NEAR the lumen
> (Submucosal, for Secretion)
> AuerBACH's is further BACK
> (between Muscles, for Motility)

What do the major salivary glands secrete?
The closer to the chin, the thicker (more mucous) the
secretion. Hence:

SUBLINGUAL > **SUBMANDIBULAR** > **PAROTID**
   (mucous)   (mixed)   (serous)

Where are basophils and B cells found?
The Blood has Basophils and B cells. The tissue
equivalents are mast cells and plasma
cells, respectively.

Which allows color vision, rods or cones?
Cones allow Color and aCuity.

MICROANATOMY AND EMBRYOLOGY QUIZ

1. Which of the following cells is not located in the central nervous system?
   a. Oligodendrocytes
   b. Neurons
   c. Schwann cells
   d. Microglia

2. Which of the following is correct regarding the thymus?
   a. It is the major source of B cells in the neonate.
   b. It is functional for thirty years in the average person.
   c. It is located in the pelvis.
   d. It is identified microscopically by the presence of Hassall bodies.

3. Bone consists of which kind of cartilage?
   a. Type 1
   b. Type 2
   c. Type 3
   d. Type 4

4. The human erythrocyte typically survives how long in the blood?
   a. 48 hours
   b. 120 days
   c. 6 months
   d. 1 year

5. Which of the following is incorrect regarding chief cells?
   a. They produce a substance that helps digest proteins.
   b. They secrete pepsin.
   c. They primarily secrete acid into the gastric lumen.
   d. They are located in the parathyroid glands.

6. Which infectious agent is not a teratogen?
   a. Cytomegalovirus (CMV)
   b. Syphilis
   c. T. gondii
   d. Chlamydia

7. Which cells make inhibin?
   a. Cells of the posterior pituitary.
   b. Cells of the adrenal cortex.
   c. Interstitial Leydig cells of the testes.
   d. Sertoli cells of the testes.

8. Which substance is not released in capacitation?
   a. Coagulase
   b. Acrosin
   c. Hyaluronidase
   d. Trypsin-like enzymes

9. When can the sex of the embryo be observed (without karyotyping)?
   a. First week
   b. Third week
   c. Fifth week
   d. Seventh week

10. Which of the following is not a derivative of the first pharyngeal arch?
    a. Muscles innervated by CN V
    b. Tensor tympani
    c. Stapedius
    d. Mylohyoid

11. Which is not a characteristic of the Tetralogy of Fallot?
    a. Displaced aorta
    b. Reduction in size of the right ventricle
    c. Narrowing of the pulmonary artery
    d. VSD

12. Which is a left-to-right heart shunt?
    a. VSD
    b. Tetralogy of Fallot
    c. Persistent truncus arteriosus
    d. Transposition of the great vessels

13. Which of the following is correct?
    a. Meissner's plexus controls motility of the gut
    b. Secretion into the lumen is influenced mainly by the activity of Auerbach's plexus
    c. Meissner's plexus is especially prominent in the tongue
    d. Auerbach's plexus is located between the circular and longitudinal layers of muscle

NEUROSCIENCE

Think of the neuron as a lollipop:
The candy part in the illustration to the right represents the cell body, which appears grey due to a lack of myelin. The white stick of the lollipop represents the axon, which is myelinated and gives the white matter its appearance.

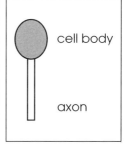

What sorts of pain do types A and C fibers carry?
Type **A** carries **A**cute stabbing pain.
Type **C** carries **C**hronic dull burning pain.

How do the sympathetics control the eye?
They let you fight or flee. If you are to take on a predator, for example, you require a widely dilated pupil so you can see everything, and you need to adjust for far-vision to watch for approaching predators. These effects will be important when you study pharmacology.

Which ciliary nerve contains all the parasympathetic innervation to the eye?
The short ciliary nerve is the Napoleon of the eye; although it's short, it has all the PNS power.

What occurs during the accommodation reaction?
        In aCCommodation... the eyes Converge;
        the pupils and ciliary lens muscles Constrict.

What happens when you stimulate versus infarct the frontal eye field (FEF)?
A stimulus (e.g., from seizure) to the FEF tells the eyes to look away (this is an unimportant event). A lesion to the FEF makes the eyes look towards the side of the lesion (this is an important event, so the eyes are telling you to take a look).

Do superior eye muscles intort or extort the eyeball?
Remember **SIN**:
        Superior muscles **IN**tort.

Where does CSF come from and go to?

> The Choroid plexus Creates it, and
> the Arachnoid villi Absorb it.

How do the foramina of Magendie and Luschka exit the 4th ventricle?

> Magendie is Medial
> Luschkas are Lateral

---

hat does a hemorrhage within the pons do to the pupils?
        Pons causes **P**in**P**oint **P**upils.

What are the parts of the limbic system?

Although several references disagree as to what should be included as essential to the system, the following mnemonic is fairly reliable:

CATS Love **HAM**:

> **C**ingulate gyrus
> **A**nterior Thalamus
> **S**eptal area
> **L**imbic lobe
> **H**ippocampus
> **A**mygdala
> **M**amillary bodies

HAM sounds like hand, which is part of the limb (which sounds like limbic).

What are the functions of the limbic system?

It controls the **5 F's**: **F**eed, **F**eel (emotions), **F**ight, **F**light, **F**ornicate.

What are the components of the Papez circuit?

MATCH

> **M**amillary
> **A**nterior Thalamus
> **C**ingulate
> **H**ippocampus

What parts of the thalamus control hunger?
The lateral and medial parts act like the pterygoids
(see page 8). Stimulating the LATERAL thalamus
stimulates hunger (the LATERAL pterygoids open the
mouth). Stimulating the MEDIAL thalamus stimulates
satiety (the MEDIAL pterygoids close the mouth).
The opposites are true for destructive lesions of the
two areas.

---

*What are the fasciculus gracilis and fasciculus
cuneatus?*
These contain dorsal column fibers.

> **Gracilis** is for **grace**fulness (innervates the legs)
> **Cun**eatus is for **cunning** (innervates the upper
> body, closer to the cunning mind)

How does Guillain-Barre present?
"Bottoms-up!" Paralysis of the legs, moving upwards.

What do VPL and VPM receive?
VPL gets sensation from the Limbs.
VPM gets taste from the Mouth.

What is Romberg's sign?
When the patient closes his eyes, he **ROAMS** (sways)
with **ROM**berg's sign.

How do you identify the levels of the brainstem in section?

The **MIDBRAIN**. Look for the red nucleus medially and substantia nigra laterally:

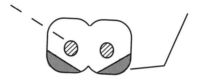

The **PONS**. Look for CN 7 running circles around CN 6. If not present, exclude other layers.

The **MEDULLA**. Look for the inferior olives:

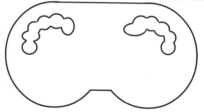

What are the lobes of the cerebellum?

- The **A**nterior lobe which gets the **A**scending pathways and is destroyed by **A**lcoholism.
- The **D**orsal lobe which gives the **D**escending pathways.
- The vestibular feeds the flocculonodular.

To where does the vermis project?
"Vermis" means worm, so think of a **FAST** worm, since the vermis projects to the **FAST**igial nucleus.

What are the inhibitory and stimulatory fibers of the cerebellum?
EVERYTHING is INHIBITORY except the entering fibers (climbing and mossy) and the granules (which give parallel fibers).

What are the roles of the fastigial, the interposed, and the dentate nuclei?
- The **fastigial**, located in the *center,* affects balance down the *midline* of the body.
- The **interposed**, located *laterally,* affect limb proprioception (i.e., *lateral* balance).
- The **dentate** (i.e., teeth-like) gives the cerebellum some teeth, since with it the cerebellum can do more than simply balance; the dentate nucleus helps initiate, plan, and time movement.

Lesions to the cerebellar cortex present with IPSILATERAL lesions. This is in contrast to lesions of the cerebral cortex, which present with CONTRALATERAL lesions.

What is caloric nystagmus?
COWS:
- If you put **C**old water in the ear, the nystagmus is towards the **O**pposite direction.
- If you put **W**arm water in the ear, the nystagmus is towards the **S**ame direction.

What do the two salivatory nuclei control?

- The SUPERIOR nucleus contributes to all the salivatory and lacrimal glands except the parotid. CN 7 is involved.
- The INFERIOR nucleus contributes to the parotid gland via the otic ganglion and CN 9.

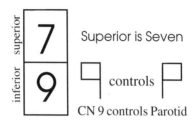

What ganglia control the parotids?
The ***par-o-tids*** run off a ***pair-of-otics*** (otic ganglia).

What part of the substantia nigra is affected in Parkinson's disease?
The **PAR**s **COM**pacta is involved in Parkinson's (i.e., **PARCOM**son's disease).

Where is norepinephrine primarily made in the brain?
Too much NE overstimulates the sympathetic nervous system and makes you **LOCO** (crazy). Hence, it is found mainly in the **LOCUS** ceruleus. Serotonin, which makes you sleepy, is found in the raphe nucleus.

What are the divisions of the CN V sensory nucleus?
Their locations in the cord represent their evolutionary advances, where the lowest part is primitive and the highest part is evolved.

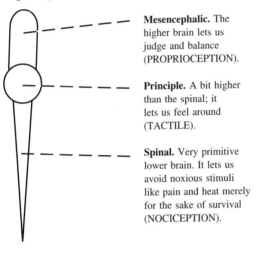

Mesencephalic. The higher brain lets us judge and balance (PROPRIOCEPTION).

Principle. A bit higher than the spinal; it lets us feel around (TACTILE).

Spinal. Very primitive lower brain. It lets us avoid noxious stimuli like pain and heat merely for the sake of survival (NOCICEPTION).

What does the supraoptic nucleus (SON) do?
Standing in the SUN, the SON is stimulated to release ADH and hence to help the body conserve water.

What nucleus controls the circadian rhythm?
The SCN (suprachiasmatic nucleus) controls it, and almost looks like an abbreviation of circadian (i.e.: SirCadiaN).

What is decortical and decerebrate rigidity?
- Since the cortical area is in the *higher* brain, the arms are flexed *up*.
- The decerebrate lesion is in the *lower* brain, so the arms are extended *down*.

Which nerve wraps around the brainstem from posterior, crossing the midline before exiting?
CN IV. Recall that CN FOUR lets you look at your FORE*arm* (page 6). Similarly, CN 4 hugs the brainstem like a pair of *arms*. This is a unique characteristic.

What nucleus innervates the uvula?
The nucleus ambig**UU**s innervates the **U**v**U**la (and the pharynx and larynx).

How do lesions of CN 11 and 12 present?
- CN 11 damage *faces the lesion*. You can't look away from the lesion.
- CN 12 damage *licks the lesion*. The tongue deviates ipsilateral when protruded.

What does the auditory pathway consist of?
E. COLI (as in the bug)...

> **E**ighth nerve
>
> **C**ochlear nerve
> **O**livary nucleus (i.e., superior)
> **L**ateral lemniscus
> **I**nferior colliculus

NEUROSCIENCE QUIZ

1. Which of the following is a property of the eye?
   a. Sympathetic innervation permits accommodation.
   b. A lesion of the left frontal eye field would present with eye deviation to the right.
   c. A lesion of the long ciliary nerve would reduce the ability of the ipsilateral eye to constrict.
   d. The superior oblique muscle can intort the eye.

For questions 2-4, match the following:
   a. Foramen of Luschka
   b. Choroid plexus
   c. Both
   d. Neither

2. CSF synthesis

3. Lesion of this may cause hydrocephalus.

4. Permits escape of CSF from the fourth ventricle caudally.

5. Which is not associated with the limbic system?
   a. Amygdala
   b. Cingulate gyrus
   c. Supraoptic nucleus
   d. Anterior thalamic nucleus

6. Which is true regarding the spinal cord?
   a. It sends most of its proprioceptive fibers to the VPM.
   b. Lesions to the fasciculus gracilis would affect proprioception from the biceps brachii.
   c. Complete transection at T7 would terminate respiration.
   d. Hemisection at T9 would spare the fasciculus cuneatus.

7. Which is true regarding the cerebellum?
   a. Climbing fibers are stimulatory.
   b. Lesion to the right cortex affects the left side, primarily.
   c. Proprioceptive sensation is mainly received by the dorsal lobe.
   d. The vermis, which projects to the fastigial nucleus, is responsible for smooth limb movement.

8. Which is correct?
   a. The superior salivatory nucleus affects the otic ganglia.
   b. Stimulating the inferior salivatory nucleus causes parotid serous secretion.
   c. CN 7 is associated with the inferior salivatory nucleus.
   d. Ablation of the inferior salivatory nucleus may end the ability to cry.

For questions 9-16, match the one correct answer with each function:
   a. Spinal nucleus of CN V
   b. Suprachiasmatic nucleus
   c. CN XI nucleus
   d. Pars compacta of the substantia nigra
   e. Septal nucleus
   f. Locus ceruleus
   g. Raphe nucleus
   h. Lateral thalamus
   i. Supraoptic nucleus
   j. Mesencephalic nucleus of CN V
   k. Medial thalamus
   l. Nucleus ambiguus
   m. Nucleus solitarius

9. Ablation causes hunger

10. Ablation causes inadequate response to hypovolemia

11. Stimulation causes elevation of the uvula

12. Stimulation causes satiety

13. A bee sting to the face is transmitted to this structure

14. Lacks dopamine in Parkinson's disease

15. Main storage site of norepinephrine

16. Permits the circadian rhythm

For questions 17 and 18, choose the correct answer:
   a. Tongue deviates left when protruded
   b. Tongue deviates right when protruded
   c. Both
   d. Neither

17. A lower motor neuron lesion

18. A lesion to the right CN 12

BIOCHEMISTRY

What are the collagen synthesis defects?

Scurvy   •   prolyl hydroxylase

CONE $\Biggl\{$ **C**-terminal cleavage defect is **O**steogenesis imperfecta; **N**-terminal cleavage defect is **E**hlers-Danlos

Lathyrism
*(Marfan's
syndrome)*   •   lysyl oxidase

How does the number of prolines influence collagen stability?
PROLINE is **PRO-LINK**.
Increasing the number of prolines will increase the stability of collagen at higher temperatures.

What are exons and introns?
EXons **EX**press, while **INT**rons **INT**erfere.

What is the start codon?
AUG, as in you start school in **AUG**ust.

When are glucagon and insulin released?
When **GLUC**ose is **GONE**, bring out **GLUC**a**GON**.
To get glucose **IN** to cells, bring out **IN**sul**IN**.

What do maltose, sucrose and lactose contain?

- **MALTOSE** is simply two glucoses.

- To obtain **SUCROSE**, the S can be converted to a G and then an F:

SUCROSE is GLUCOSE
plus SRUCTOSE
(GLUCOSE plus FRUCTOSE)

- **LACTOSE** is **GLUCOSE** plus **gaLACTOSE**

How do mannose and galactose differ from glucose?

Starting with glucose:

$$H_2COH$$
$$H\ COH$$

3rd Carbon: ┌─────────────┐
              │ HO CH   │
              └─────────────┘

$$H\ COH$$
$$H\ COH$$
$$H_2COH$$

GLUCOSE

The symbol for a MAN has the lines ABOVE the circle...

Similarly, the OH switch of MANnose is ABOVE that of glucose:

H₂COH

2nd Carbon: | HOCH |

H COH

H COH

H COH

H₂COH

MANNOSE

The symbol for a GAL (woman) has the lines BELOW the circle...

♀

Similarly, the OH switch of GALactose is BELOW that of glucose:

H₂COH

H COH

H COH

4th Carbon: | HOCH |

H COH

H₂COH

GALACTOSE

What are some of the lysosomal storage diseases?

Remember *ANUS:*

alpha-g**A**l**A**ctosidase deficiency	F**A**bry's disease
s**Phi**N**gomyelinase deficiency	**N**iemann-**P**ick's disease
gl**U**cocerebrosidase deficiency	Ga**U**cher's disease
hexo**S**aminidase deficiency (sounds like taysachsaminidase)	Tay-**S**achs disease

Outline of the Citric Acid Cycle:

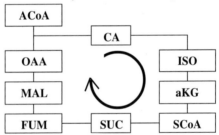

Abbreviations:
ACoA = Acetyl CoA; CA = Citric Acid;
ISO = Isocitrate; aKG = alpha-Ketoglutarate;
SCoA = Succinyl CoA; SUC = Succinate;
FUM = Fumerate; MAL = Malate;
OAA = Oxaloacetic Acid

Note:
1. This cycle moves clockwise.
2. NADH or FADH$_2$ is made prior to a corner. Hence, one is made prior to SCoA, FUM, and

OAA. In addition, one is made prior to aKG.

3. FADH$_2$ is made prior to Fumerate only (associate the F's), whereas the other reactions produce NADH.

4. NADH or FADH$_2$-producing steps involve dehydrogenases.

5. The order of metabolites can be recalled with the following:

The cycle begins with the reaction of acetyl CoA and OAA to make CITRIC ACID, hence the name of this cycle. The upper right corner of this box represents a transient intermediate (cis-aconitate) and the conversion of CITRATE to isoCITRATE. The cycle then enters a complex very similar to the one that produces ACoA from pyruvate; if you know the pyruvate dehydrogenase complex, you know the aKG dehydrogenase complex. Instead of acetyl CoA, this complex gives rise to SUCCINYL CoA. SCoA gives up the CoA to become plain old SUCCINATE, and in so doing gives rise to GTP.

When you study this cycle, first you say: "This SUCKS! (succinate)." Then you get so pissed off, you're FUMING (fumerate). Finally, you start doing MALICIOUS deeds (malate). Malate is converted to OAA, and the cycle is over.

Needless to say, this much-touted pathway seldom arises in clinical medicine.

What are the electron transport system inhibitors?

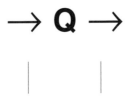

Rotenone   Antimycin-A

All the popular ones (cyanide, H_2S, and carbon monoxide) act on the very last step, where oxygen accepts the electrons.

What are the inhibitors of the ATP-ADP translocase?
This translocase moves energy equivalents from one side of the mitochondrial membrane to the other.
The names of the inhibitors reflect this.

ATRACTYLOSIDE	Attract to the other side
bongKREKIC acid	A cricket that hops to the other side

What is Glycerol-3-Phosphate (G3P) dehydrogenase?
This reaction is seen when:
1. glycerol enters glycolysis / gluconeogenesis;
2. fat cells make triglycerides from glycerol;
3. reducing potential is transported into the mitochondria from glycolysis to the electron transport chain.

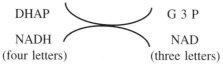

DHAP		G 3 P
NADH		NAD
(four letters)		(three letters)

What are the first enzymes of gluconeogenesis?

PEACE and **PEPSI**

1. **Pea**C**e** (**PC** is **P**yruvate **C**arboxylase)
2. **Pepsi** (**PEP-C** is **PEP C**arboxylase)
This is in contrast to the last step of glycolysis, pyruvate kinase.

What does transketolase do and what cofactor is involved?
• Transke**TO**lase moves **TWO**-carbon units.
• Transaldolase moves 3-C units.

Where is LCAT?
LCAT is in the **L**ipoprotein,
unlike ACAT which is in the tissue.

How are amino acids arranged in a polypeptide?

AmiNo aCids go from N-terminal to C-terminal

What are the essential amino acids?
Vice-President Milt (**VP MILT**):

> **V**aline
> **P**henylalanine
>
> **M**ethionine
> **I**soleucine
> **L**eucine and **L**ycine
> **T**hreonine and **T**ryptophan
> (and in PKU, Tyrosine)

What are the structures of serine and threonine?
SERINE is serene, since it has alcohol.
THREonine has THREE different groups
    (alcohol, hydrogen, and a methyl).

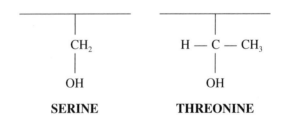

What are the branched-chain amino acids?
They LIVe, but the MSUD patients do not.
Maple Syrup Urine Disease (MSUD) is due to a defect in metabolism of branched-chain amino acids, and commonly causes neonatal death.

> **L**eucine
> **I**soleucine
> **V**aline

These can be used to remember what amino acids are ketogenic, which are glucogenic, and which are both...

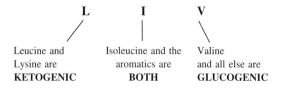

L	**I**	**V**
Leucine and Lysine are **KETOGENIC**	Isoleucine and the aromatics are **BOTH**	Valine and all else are **GLUCOGENIC**

What are the roles of SAM (S-adenosylmethionine)?
Sam is a Mellow Cretin who teaches P.E. (physical education):

Mellow	Melatonin formation
Cretin	Creatine formation
P	Phosphatidylcholine formation
E	Epinephrine formation

SAM is involved in this cycle:

M is Methionine
H is Homocysteine
This cycle goes clockwise.

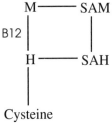

SAM is also seen here:

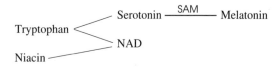

What do the carboxypeptidases cleave?

- Carboxypeptidase **A** cleaves off **A**romatics from the C-terminal.
- Carboxypeptidase **B** cleaves off **B**asic amino acids from the C-terminal.

Arrange the purines and pyrimidines:
First, arrange them in alphabetical order: Adenosine, Cytosine, Guanosine, Thymine, Uracil.
Now, reorganize as follows:

Notice that the p**Y**rimidines are c**Y**tosine and th**Y**midine (and in RNA, uracil).

Also note the purine and pyrimidine rings are always numbered starting at the aspartate or glycine nitrogen, moving towards the glutamine nitrogen.

How are purines and pyrimidines made?
- PURINES are derived from iNOSINate, because when you're PURE you know NO SIN.
- On the other hand, PYRIMIDINES are not so pure. They are derived from OROTIC acid since they're EROTIC. Orotic acid is converted to UMP, since they hUMP.

*What do Uracil synthesis (i.e., pyrimidine synthesis)
and the Urea cycle have in common?*
Besides having the same first letter, they have similar
first reactions:

Urea:	*Uracil:*
• in the mitochondria	• in the cytosol
• via CPS I	• via CPS II
• NAG stimulates	• NAG won't stimulate
• NH_4^+ is the donor	• glutamine is the donor

(CPS = Carbamoyl Phosphate Synthetase)

---

*What is the main stimulator of the urea cycle's
first step?*
N-AcetylGlutamate (NAG) *nags* the cycle to take out
the trash (urea and CO_2 waste).

---

*How is the adrenal cortex arranged and what does
each layer secrete?*

From outside to in, the zonae spell GFR, as in Glomerular Filtration Rate *(see renal physiology)*:	...in this order, the hormones they produce spell ACT:
Glomerulosa **F**asciculata **R**eticularis	**A**ldosterone **C**ortisol **T**estosterone

ALdosterone is the same as minerALcorticoids, while
CORTIsol is the same as CORTIcosteroids. The
androgens made by the reticularis include testosterone
and very little estrogen.

Which of the cortical hormones are protein bound?

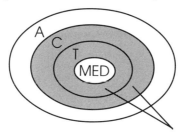

The two layers that make CORTISOL and TESTOSTERONE can be considered "bound" to the adrenal medulla, unlike the zona glomerulosa (which makes aldosterone). In this way, we can remember that cortisol and testosterone are also bound to protein in serum, while aldosterone is not.

When recalling the enzymes that act on these three cortical hormones, draw this scheme:

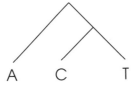

This can be redrawn with the points where enzyme deficiencies would block indicated:

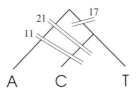

What are the fat-soluble vitamins?

FAKED: The **F**at-solubles are **A**, **K**, **E**, and **D**.

What are the functions of Vitamin B6?

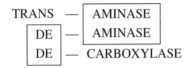

What are the metabolites that form cholesterol (in order)?

A	**A**cetyl CoA
Handsome	**H**MG CoA
Man	**M**evalonate
Is	**I**sopentenyl pyrophosphate (PP)
Good	**G**eranyl PP
For	**F**arnesyl PP
Sex,	**S**qualene
Love, and	**L**anosterol
Cuddling	**C**holesterol

BIOCHEMISTRY QUIZ

1. Which is *not* due to a defect in collagen?
   a. Ehlers-Danlos syndrome
   b. Scurvy
   c. Rickets
   d. Osteogenesis imperfecta

2. Which is matched correctly?
   a. Maltose is two fructose molecules
   b. Galactose is glucose plus lactose
   c. Sucrose is fructose plus glucose
   d. Fructose is sucrose plus deoxyhemoglobin

For questions 3-6, match the correct disease with the enzyme deficiency:
   a. Gaucher's
   b. Fabry's
   c. Felty's
   d. Niemann-Pick's
   e. Tay-Sachs

3. Sphingomyelinase deficiency

4. Alpha-galactosidase deficiency

5. Hexosaminidase deficiency

6. Glucocerebrosidase deficiency

7. Which step in the TCA cycle makes $FADH_2$?
   a. Citrate synthase
   b. Fumerase
   c. Fumerate dehydrogenase
   d. Malate dehydrogenase

8. Which is not an enzyme in gluconeogenesis?
   a. Pyruvate carboxylase
   b. PEP carboxylase
   c. Glucose 6-phosphatase
   d. Pyruvate kinase

9. Which is not an essential amino acid?
   a. Glycine
   b. Leucine
   c. Phenylalanine
   d. Isoleucine

10. Which is correct?
   a. Leucine is both keto and glucogenic.
   b. Valine is ketogenic.
   c. Tyrosine is both keto and glucogenic.
   d. Lysine is glucogenic.

11. Which is produced using S-adenosylmethionine?
   a. Melatonin
   b. Melanin
   c. Phosphatidylinositol
   d. Tryptophan

12. Which is correct?

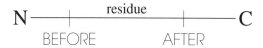

a. Chemotrypsin cleaves before leucine residues.
b. Carboxypeptidase A cleaves after aromatic amino acids.
c. Carboxypeptidase A cleaves after basic amino acids.
d. Carboxypeptidase B cleaves before the above residue.

13. Which is not correct?
   a. Adenosine is a purine.
   b. Purines are derived from inosinate.
   c. Inosinate gives rise to orotic acid.
   d. Orotic acid gives rise to UMP.

14. Which is correct?
   a. The zona glomerulosa secretes cortisol.
   b. The zona that produces testosterone contains 21-hydroxylase.
   c. Aldosterone is mostly protein-bound.
   d. The product of the zona reticularis is protein-bound.

15. Which is a water-soluble vitamin?
   a. A
   b. B
   c. D
   d. E

For questions 16-20, match the one correct answer to each item:
   a. Urea cycle
   b. Uracil synthesis
   c. Both
   d. Neither

16. Stimulated by high levels of N-acetylglutamate.

17. Occurs in the nucleus.

18. Glutamate is the donor of nitrogen.

19. Uses CPS I.

20. Permits RNA synthesis.

21. Which is a correct sequence in cholesterol synthesis?
   a. Squalene, Lanosterol, Cholesterol
   b. Acetyl CoA, Mevalonate, HMG CoA
   c. Geranyl PP, Squalene, Cholesterol
   d. Mevalonate, HMG CoA, Squalene

PHYSIOLOGY

What are the roles of FSH and LH?
FSH gets you onto the diving board (puts the shuttle on the launch pad; loads the gun):
- In men it *produces* sperm (which are like little fish [FSH]);
- In women it *produces* ova.

LH jumps you off the diving board (ignites the fuel; shoots the gun):
- In men it causes the *release* of testosterone (acts on Leydig cells [see page 28])
- In women it causes the *release* of ova.

What is the role of the pineal gland?
The pineal gland regulates melatonin and scrotonin release. While melanin is associated with *being* dark, melatonin is *released* in the dark and delays sexual maturation.
- The **D**ark **D**oesn't let you mature into puberty; it **D**elays sexual onset.
- The **L**ight **L**ets you mature into puberty, lowers melatonin, and causes precocious puberty.

Which is better, T_4 or T_3?
Although T_3 has more activity in the periphery, T_4 wins out everywhere else. T_4 is released more from the thyroid, is in a four-fold higher level in the blood, is more protein-bound, and has a greater half-life. Hence, T_4 is "better."

What is the formula for renal clearance?

$$\text{Clearance} = \frac{UV}{P}$$

Clearance means *you've peed*:

> You've = **UV** (urine concentration x volume of urine)
> Peed = **P** (plasma concentration)

What is the ferrous iron form and is it normal in hemoglobin?

> "Just the Two of Us"
> Fe^{+2} is ferroUS
> (Fe^{+3} is ferric)

The TWO form occurs in US normally. When hemoglobin contains the three form of iron, it cannot bind oxygen (such as in nitrite poisoning).

Where are the hot and cold receptors in the brain?
The hot and the cold receptors are located in the anterior and posterior thalamus regions respectively.

> Hot and cold is front and back.

Two important formulae are:

> PRT (that is, P x R = T)   *"Pretty*
> PQR (that is, P = Q x R)   *Pucker"*

where:

> **P** is Pressure   **Q** is Flow
> **R** is Resistance   **T** is wall Tension

What are the signs of heart failure?

A B C D E

> **A**cidosis
> **B**lue skin
> **C**old skin
> **D**ilated heart
> **E**dema

How do insulin and calcitonin act?
They keep things IN the tissue and out of the blood:

> Insul**IN** keeps it (glucose) **IN**
> Calciton**IN** keeps it (calcium) **IN**

What is the role of renin?

> Renin stops the runnin'

Since *renin* release ultimately causes water retention, you don't *run* to the bathroom as often.

Where in the brain is GnRH made?
Gono**RH**ea is a **MEAN** bugger:
   The **M**edian **E**minence of the **A**rcuate **N**ucleus

---

What overall adrenergic affinity does epinephrine versus NE have?

BEAN

> **B**eta is preferred by
> **E**pinephrine;
> **A**lpha is preferred by
> **N**orepinephrine.

Which adrenergic receptors do epinephrine and norepinephrine (NE) stimulate?
EPI does EVERYthing, NOR does NOT. Epinephrine covers both alpha-1 and -2, and beta-1 and -2. NE does not stimulate beta-2.

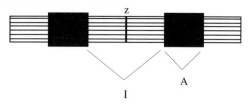

How do sympathetics alter insulin and renin release?

(alpha 1)	lowers nothing
ALPHA 2	lowers Insulin
BETA 1	raises Renin
BETA 2	raises Insulin

How do sympathetics alter fat and glucose metabolism?

$$\begin{aligned} &\qquad\qquad\text{BETA 1} = \text{LIPOLYSIS} \\ &\text{GLYCOGENOLYSIS} = \text{BETA 2} \\ &\qquad\qquad\text{BETA 3} = \text{LIPOLYSIS} \end{aligned}$$

Note that beta-blocking drugs may affect beta 2, thus lowering blood glucose.

What's another name for a widened (dilated) pupil?
MYDRIASIS means WIDE-IRISES. Miosis is pin-point (constricted) pupil.

What do alpha and beta stimulation do to blood vessels?

Alpha Constrict while Beta Dilate vessels:

| A | B | = | Alpha | Beta |
| C | D | | Constrict | Dilate |

What do alpha and beta stimulation do to the eye?
Alpha (A) widens the pupil. Beta (B) widens the lens.

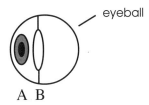

A B

Remember, sympathetic stimulation enables you to spot distant predators in a fight-or-flight situation. Hence, the eyes widen.

What is the connection between insulin, glucagon, and somatostatin?
Somato*statin* causes *stasis* of hormone release, so it inhibits release of both insulin and glucagon. Glucagon is the opposite of somatostatin, as it *stimulates* release of both somatostatin and insulin. Insulin is a mean dictator, who stops glucagon release, and doesn't even bother with somatostatin.

Here is a very quick method of determining whether someone is alkalotic or acidotic. First look at the pH as indicated in an arterial blood gas (ABG) test (>7.4 is basic, <7.4 is acidic), then read the bicarb value:

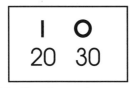

10 20 30   rewritten as...

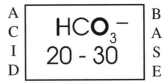

The HCO_3^- disturbance tells you this is metabolic (CO_2 disturbance indicates respiratory). Anything *less* than 20 mm Hg of bicarb indicates acidosis, anything *above* 30 mm Hg bicarb indicates alkalosis. This is particularly useful in uncompensated states.

pH < 7.4 and bicarb < 20 metabolic acidosis
pH > 7.4 and bicarb > 30 metabolic alkalosis

If the ABG deviates from this simple pattern, you will have to use another method to figure it out.

PHYSIOLOGY QUIZ

1. Which is true concerning FSH?
   a. It stimulates the production of sperm.
   b. It stimulates the release of sperm.
   c. It inhibits the production of ova.
   d. It stimulates the release of ova.

2. Which is incorrect about T_4?
   a. It has a longer half-life than T_3.
   b. It is more protein-bound than T_3.
   c. It is more prevalent in plasma than T_3.
   d. It is more active in tissues than T_3.

3. Flow through a blood vessel is doubled while resistance is tripled. The pressure is thus...
   a. Increased 4-fold
   b. Raised by half
   c. Increased 6-fold
   d. Lowered by 2/3

4. Which is incorrect?
   a. Insulin causes glucose to move into cells.
   b. Calcitonin causes calcium to stay in bones.
   c. Renin causes water to stay in the body.
   d. Melatonin causes melanin to stay in melanocytes.

For questions 5-13, choose from answers a-d:
   a. Alpha receptor
   b. Beta receptor
   c. Both
   d. Neither

5. Stimulated by norepinephrine

6. Stimulated by epinephrine

7. Epinephrine has a higher affinity for it

8. Raises insulin level

9. Lowers renin level

10. Stimulates lipolysis

11. When located on a blood vessel, its inhibition causes dilation

12. Eye-drops that induce mydriasis stimulate it

13. Eye-drops that blur vision stimulate it

14. A patient presents with recent onset (1 hour ago) of acid-base disturbance. Her ABG's (arterial blood gases) are as follows:

pH	7.30
pCO_2	35
pO_2	97.2
HCO_3	18

This patient suffers from:
a. Metabolic acidosis
b. Metabolic alkalosis
c. Respiratory acidosis
d. Respiratory alkalosis

BEHAVIORAL SCIENCES

What are Wernicke's and Broca's aphasias?
When you pronounce "WERnicke" your mouth is open, so you are capable of expressing. Hence the defect lies in comprehension (a sensory aphasia). When you pronounce "Broca" your mouth stays closed with the B, so this is an inability to express verbally (a motor aphasia).

Don't confuse Wernicke's aphasia with Wernicke-Korsakoff disease, which consists of...

WErnickE's Encephalitis
KorsaKoff's Confabulation

What are Piaget's developmental stages?

1. Sensorimotor   •   *First a person must learn the basics: sensation and motor*

2. Preoperative   •   *Preparing to operate*

3. Concrete Operative   •   *Formal is last. You dress up formally when you attend your school*

4. Formal Operative   *graduation. Likewise, a person graduates from development by passing the formal stage.*

What are the ages of Eriksonian and Freudian childhood stages?
The increments in years are achieved by multiplying by two:

    0 - 1½
    1½ - 3   (1½ x 2 = 3)
    3 - 6   (3 x 2 = 6)
    6 - 12   (6 x 2 = 12)

What are the I.Q. levels of mental retardation?
Think of angles: 30°, 45°, and 60°:

    60 ± 10 Mild
    45 ± 10 Moderate
    30 ± 10 Severe
    <20   Profound

What do alpha and beta mean in generating hypotheses?
Just remember alpha and beta as "TRUE or FALSE."

    alpha   TRUE   *that is, reject when TRUE*
    beta   FALSE *that is, accept when FALSE*

What are Bleuler's 4A's of schizophrenia?

    Autism
    Affective disorder
    Associative disorder
    Ambivalence

What does the mental status exam consist of?

ARTS & MAJIC

Appearance
Rapport
Thought process and content
Speech

Mood
Affect
Judgement
Insight
Cognition *(see below)*

What are the risk factors for suicide?

SAD PERSONS

Sex (males more successful)
Age (teens and elderly)
Depression

Prior attempts at suicide
Employment (jobless)
Recent stressors
Schizophrenia / mental illness
Organic disease
Note written
Substance abuse

How do you test a patient's cognition?

COMA

| **C**onsciousness |
| **O**rientation |
| **M**emory |
| **A**ttention |

BEHAVIORAL SCIENCES QUIZ

1. The ability to speak but not comprehend what is being said is called:
   a. Broca's aphasia
   b. Wernicke's aphasia
   c. Anosmia
   d. Wernicke-Korsakoff syndrome

2. A patient with an I.Q. of 45 is considered:
   a. Mildly retarded
   b. Moderately retarded
   c. Severely retarded
   d. Profoundly retarded

3. Which has not been considered a defining feature of schizophrenia?
   a. Inappropriate affect
   b. Autistic behavior
   c. Anosognosia
   d. Lack of rational associations in thought

4. A cognitive exam should test for all except:
   a. I.Q.
   b. Clouding of consciousness
   c. Distractibility and attention span
   d. Orientation to location

5. A major risk factor for completed suicide includes:
   a. Age of 35
   b. Black female
   c. College-graduate, recently discharged from hospital for psychotic break-down
   d. Being happily married

See the pharmacology section for drugs used in psychiatry.

PATHOLOGY

What are the leading causes of death in infancy and childhood?
CRAM (in this order of incidence):

in infancy	*in childhood*
1. **C**ongenital disease	1. **A**ccidents
2. **R**espiratory disease	2. **M**alignancy

Which occurs first: malformations or deformations?
They occur in order of M.D.:
Malformation is faulty formation of an organ, while **D**eformation occurs after the organ has developed.

How does malignancy progress from premalignancy?
Like a doctor from a medical student... M.D.:

> first, **M**etaplasia
> then, **D**ysplasia

How does Hodgkin's versus non-Hodgkin's lymphoma present?
Hodgkin is a proper fellow, so his lymphoma is localized to one spot, contiguous, and not extranodal.
Non-Hodgkin's lymphoma is typically a mess: multiple nodes involved, noncontiguous, and extranodal.

What do Auer rods indicate?
        "I see Auer rods, and that ain't all..."
You never see Auer rods with **ALL** (**A**cute **L**ymphocytic **L**eukemia); they appear in myelogenous leukemia.

Where are Flexner-Weinsteiner and Homer-Wright rosettes prominent?
HOMER is RIGHT (i.e., he knows the answer) because he studies his NEURO (neuroblastoma). In contrast, Flexner-Weinsteiner is seen mostly in retinoblastoma.

What's the difference between anasarca and ascites?
aSCITEs is in a particular SITE, the abdomen; anasarca is generalized.

Which murmurs are heard in diastole and systole?

> dIAstolic murmurs include **AI**

AI = Aortic Insufficiency
AS = Aortic Stenosis
MI = Mitral Insufficiency
MS = Mitral Stenosis

If you know this, you will remember that diastolic murmurs are AI and MS.
...Systolic murmurs, thus, must be AS and MI:

dIAstolic	AI	MS
systolic	AS	MI

What ventricle is affected by a heart attack?
The left ventricle, regardless of the coronary vessel occluded.

1. Anterior descending branch of the left coronary will damage the anterior LEFT heart
2. Circumflex of left coronary will damage the lateral LEFT heart
3. Even the right coronary will damage the posterior LEFT heart

---

What are stable and Prinzmetal's angina?

- *Stable* angina occurs when you're at work in the *stable*, and feel DEPRESSED at having such a lowly job. Hence, the ECG shows DEPRESSED ST segments.
- *Prinz*metal's angina occurs when you're a *prince* and are ELEVATED onto a throne. Here, the ST segments are ELEVATED.

What heart valves are most affected by systemic disease?
The LEFT AV valves are affected in rheumatic heart disease, SLE, and infective heart disease. The exceptions to this rule are the two disease states that affect the RIGHT AV valve: heroin abuse and carcinoid syndrome.

How do you find hemoglobin (Hg) and hematocrit (Hct) levels in a patient, given only RBC count?

$$RBC \times 3 = Hg$$
$$Hg \times 3 = Hct$$

What is Homan's sign?
HUMANS can show HOMAN's because they walk on their LEGS. Hence, this sign indicates a problem in the legs (specifically a deep vein thrombus).

The classic descriptions of emphysema and chronic bronchitis are as follows:

> A person with emPhysema is a Pink Puffer
> A person with chronic Bronchitis is a Blue Bloater

What is Plummer-Vinson?
When your IRON pipes are clogged, you call a PLUMBER. Similarly, the clogging of the esophagus with webs is due to IRON deficiency; this is characteristic of PLUMMER-Vinson.

What is Peutz-Jagher syndrome?
Mick JAGGER has Peutz-JAGHER. The singer has famous LIPS; the syndrome affects the LIPS as well, but also presents with poLYPS.

> Lips and polyps disease

What is pellagra?
Niacin deficiency, which presents with the 3 D's:

> **D**ermatitis
> **D**iarrhea
> **D**ementia

Who gets Whipple's disease?
Mr. Whipple, the guy who doesn't squeeze the Charmin. The disease is more frequent among older white men, and causes GI upset, among several other symptoms.

What blood assays are used for colon and prostate cancers?

> **P**rostate cancer shows high **PSA**.
> **C**olon cancer shows high **CEA**.

Which has a higher tendency towards malignancy: villous or tuberous colon adenoma?

VILLOUS are VILLAINS

(they are more likely premalignant).

What is absorbed mainly by the terminal ileum?
The 2 B's:

Bile and Vitamin **B**12

Who gets gall stones of the mixed or pure cholesterol types?
Classically (although not necesarilly in practice), the risk factors are as follows:

The 4 C's	The 4 F's
Cystic fibrosis	**F**at
Crohn's disease	**F**emale
Clofibrate therapy	**F**ertile
Contraceptive use	**F**orty years old or more

What are the diseases of hyperbilirubinemia?
- Most are Direct (= Conjugated; the first letters are consonants).
- A few are Indirect (= Unconjugated; the first letters are vowels). For example:
  Crigler-Najjar: (the liver says, "I don't know what language that is, so I can't conjugate you.")
  Gilbert's: (Melissa Gilbert of *Little House on the Prairie* can't get into her house, just as bilirubin can't enter the liver; thus it winds up unconjugated in the blood).

The two strange forms of conjugated hyper-bilirubinemia are Dubin-Johnson and Rotor's disease. Rotor produces a regular-colored liver, whereas Dubin-Johnson colors the liver black. Remember this as **R**otor's is **R**egular-colored; while **D**ubin-Johnson's is **D**ark-colored.

How does Budd-Chiari differ from Arnold-Chiari?
The liver starts off embryologically as a BUD, so BUDD-Chiari affects the liver. Arnold-Chiari affects the brain.

What causes flapping tremor?
Hepatic "flapatic" encephalopathy. This may be due to alcoholic cirrhosis but is not the same as delirium tremens.

What is a pinguecula versus a pterygium of the eye?
A PINGuecula makes a PING-pong ball-shaped lesion, whereas the pterygium makes a wing-shaped lesion.

What sorts of hepatic necrosis are there?

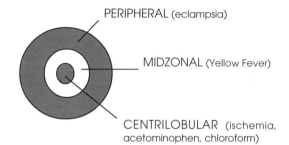

PERIPHERAL (eclampsia)

MIDZONAL (Yellow Fever)

CENTRILOBULAR (ischemia, acetominophen, chloroform)

Viruses are commonly focal, while chemicals are commonly massive. (The midzonal area can be colored yellow.)

What are the predisposing factors for liver and gall bladder disease?

Biliary disease occurs mostly among women.

Disease	Risk
Primary sclerosing cholangitis	Men with ulcerative colitis
Primary biliary cirrhosis	Women with Anti-Mitochondrial Antibodies (AMA)
Liver cell adenoma	Women on oral contraceptives
Angiosarcoma	Vinyl chloride, arsenic, Thorotrast
Hepatocellular carcinoma	Hepatitis B, moldy peanuts

What are the two main causes of acute pancreatitis?
Eating and drinking. A high fat diet or a big alcohol load can precipitate this disease. Trypsinogen activation is the initiating event for this disease, as well as for normal intestinal digestion.

Chronic pancreatitis is due mostly to alcohol, but also biliary tract disease.

What ages get polycystic kidney disease?
The autosomal **D**ominant form is found in a**D**ults. Children get the autosomal recessive form.

What do you look for in a urinalysis?
The 4-C's: **C**asts, **C**rystals, **C**ells, and **C**ontaminants.

What is nephrotic syndrome?
Unlike in nephr**I**tic syndrome, people with nephr**O**tic syndrome become puffy, like an **O**. They bloat because of salt water retention and protein loss.

What is Berger's disease?
Not to be confused with Buerger's disease, Berger's is pronounced Bar-jay's. The A of Barjay tells you the disease is a deposition of IgA antibodies in the mesangium of the kidney. The other disease which also deposits IgA in the mesangium is Henoch-Schonlein purpura.

What is epispadias versus hypospadias?
Epi is *uppy*-spadias (the urethra leaves ABOVE the normal position).
Hy*po* is be*low*-spadias (the urethra is BELOW the normal position).

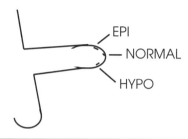

Where do you see wire-loop kidneys histologically?
LUPus shows LOOPS.

What part of the brain does herpes affect?
Scratching his temple, he thinks, "Did I sleep with her? I can't recall..." He's scratching his temple because herpes affects the TEMPORAL lobe. Of course, if he did sleep with HER, then maybe she was the one who gave him HERpes.

How does Horner's syndrome present?
Ptosis, miosis, anhidrosis

What is Meniere's disease?
Meni*ere*'s is of the *ear*. It is increased pressure of fluid in the inner ear. Mene*trier*e's is of the **t**ummy.

What is the scleroderma syndrome?

CREST	Calcinosis Raynaud's phenomenon Esophageal dysmotility Sclerodactyly Telangiectasia

---

What do you look for in diagnosing malignant melanoma?
Either ABCD or the 4-S's, whichever helps more.

ABCD	**The 4 S's**
Asymmetrical	**S**ymmetry
Border irregular	**S**hape
Color non-uniform	**S**hade
Diameter large	**S**ize

What's the difference between Hunter's and Hurler's?
In Hurler's (not Hunter's), the patient's eyes cloud up. Think of hurling (vomiting) so hard that your eyes cloud up. Otherwise put, you can't hunt well if it's cloudy.

Furthermore, hunting is a sexy sport for men, so Hunter's disease is sex-linked.

How do you identify a PKU patient?
By the musty smell...
"P—U! What an odor!" *(P—U = PKU)*

What is DiGeorge disease?
Instead of "By George, I think I've got it!" say "DiGeorge, I think I've got it!" The irony is you don't got it (a thyroid) if you have DiGeorge disease.

How does De Quervain's thyroiditis present?
With a PAINful mass, unlike other forms of thyroiditis.

> De Quer*vain* means *pain*.

What are the main causes of hyperCortisolism, hyperAldosteronism, and hyperTestosteronism?
These hormonal excesses correspond to the degrees of severity of tumor, where carcinoma is worse than adenoma which is worse than hyperplasia.

	C	hyperplasia of cortex
CAT:	**A**	adenoma of cortex
	T	carcinoma of cortex

What are the symptoms of Cushing's syndrome?
Aside from possible hypertension (due to higher aldosterone release), a patient shows the classic 6 C's of Cushing's syndrome:

> **C**ortisol elevated
> **C**ollagen synthesis reduced
> **C**alcium uptake reduced
> **C**omplexion poor (acne and hirsutism)
> **C**entripedal obesity
> **C**razy

Cushing's disease is due to high ACTH; Peter Cushing is a famous ACTor.

How do serous versus mucinous ovarian tumors present?
Serous is serious...

SEROUS
looks serious

(The pair of eyes represents the ovaries, while the pupils are the tumors. Notice the serous tumor tends to be unilocular [one lesion per ovary] and bilateral. Also notice the eyelashes, which indicate the ciliated appearance of the tumor microscopically.)

In contrast, the mucinous tumor is multilocular and unilateral:

MUCINOUS

What are the effects of sexual activity on breast, ovarian, and uterine cancers?

BO says, "Use it or lose it!"

BO = Breast and Ovarian cancers

"Use it or lose it" means a woman ought to have sex in order to prevent breast and ovarian cancers. In other words, nulliparity (not having children) and infertility are risk factors for these two forms of cancer. Similarly, oral contraceptives are believed to protect against ovarian and uterine cancers.

What is the effect of sex on cervical squamous cell carcinoma?

> **SIN** begets **CIN**

SIN = promiscuity (having many partners and having intercourse at an early age)

CIN = Cervical Intraepithelial Neoplasia

In short, the risk factors of promiscuity forementioned, in addition to oral contraceptive use, increase the risk of cervical SC carcinoma in women. The moral of the story is, have lots of kids... just don't have sex.

What are important risk factors for endometrial cancer?

LONER

> **L**ate menopause
> **O**besity
> **N**ulliparity
> **E**xogenous estrogens
> **R**adiation

What are the important masses found in the anterior mediastinum?

The four T's...

> **T**hymoma
> **T**eratoma
> **T** cell lymphoma
> **T**hyroid

What are the causes of hypercoagulable blood?
Seven things that cause **CHILLED** blood:

1.	**C**ancers
2.	**H**eparin
3.	**I**nflammatory bowel disease (UC, Crohn's)
4.	**L**eukemia
5.	**L**upus anticoagulant
6.	**E**strogens (and pregnancy)
7.	**D**eficiencies (of ATIII, proteins C & S)

Here is a list of certain chromosomal diseases:

Chromosome	Disease
4	Huntington's *(HUNT 4 Red October)*
5p del	Cri-du-chat
7	Cystic fibrosis
8, 14	Burkitt's lymphoma
9, 22	Chronic Myelogenous Leukemia
10	MEN type II
11	MEN type I, Wilm's tumor, aniridia, beta-globin defects
13 q 14	Retinoblastoma, osteoblastoma
21	Down's, Alzheimer's

Strange Associations:

These diseases may occur together:

Thymoma and **Myasthenia gravis**	**Bronchiectasis, Infertility** *(Kartagener's syndrome)*, and **Dextrocardia**
Dupuytren's contracture and **Hydronephrosis** *(due to retroperitoneal fibromatosis)*	**Ulcerative colitis, Primary sclerosing cholangitis,** and **Ankylosing spondylitis**
Polycystic kidneys and **Berry aneurysms of the circle of Willis**	

Where are the typical defects in alpha and beta thalassemias?

Alpha is due to DNA defects, beta is due to RNA defects. This order corresponds with protein synthesis (DNA is first transcribed, then RNA is translated).

A	DNA
B	RNA

What is the most common malignancy of MAJOR and minor salivary glands?

Think ACME, as in the cartoon brick company:

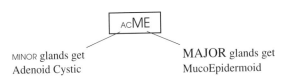

MINOR glands get Adenoid Cystic

MAJOR glands get MucoEpidermoid

These problems may indicate a certain disease:

Pancreatic disease and **Emphysema**	→	α-1-antitrypsin deficiency
Renal disease and **Lung disease**	→	Goodpasture's disease
Nose, lung, and kidney granulomas	→	Wegener's disease
Liver and brain disease, and **Corneal deposits**	→	Wilson's disease
Blond hair and **Failure to thrive**	→	PKU
Neonatal bowel obstruction and **Bronchiectasis**	→	Cystic fibrosis
Anemia and **Sensory deficits**	→	Vitamin B12 deficiency
Abnormal calcium level and **Infections**	→	DiGeorge syndrome
Enlarged testes and **Mental retardation**	→	Fragile-X syndrome
Ascites, Hydrothorax, and **Ovarian mass**	→	Meig's tumor
Clubbing, Arthritis, and **New bone growth**	→	Lung cancer
Horner's syndrome and **"Funny bone" pain**	→	Apical lung tumor

Here are some non-infectious cellular inclusions:

	Contents	Disease/ Process
Lipofuscin	Membrane lipoproteins	Aging
Basophilic stippling		Lead toxicity
Ringed sideroblasts	Mitochondria	Lead toxicity
Mallory bodies	Prekeratin filaments	Several liver diseases
Heinz bodies	Hemoglobin	glc-6-P DH deficiency
Döhle bodies	Rough ER	PMN's in severe sepsis
Toxic granulations	Azurophilic granules	PMN's in severe sepsis
Auer rods	Abnormal lyosomes	Myelogenous leukemia
Councilman bodies		Yellow fever
Russell bodies	Immunoglobins	Multiple myeloma
Hemosiderin	Ferritin	Iron excess
Neurofibrillary tangles	Cytoskeleton	Alzheimer's, Downs
Psammomma bodies	Calcium	Cancers

	Contents	**Disease/Process**
Schaumann bodies	Calcium	Sarcoidosis
Aschoff bodies	Fibrinoid necrosis	Acute rheumatic fever
Zebra bodies		Lysosomal storage disease

Some Famous Antibodies:

AMA (anti-mitochondrial Ab)	Primary biliary cirrhosis
ANCA (anti-neutrophil cytoplasm Ab)	RPGN with no etiology
Anti-dsDNA Ab	SLE
Anti-ssDNA or anti-protein Ab	Rheumatoid arthritis

How do pheochromocytomas present?
The 10% rule applies:

> 10% are extra-adrenal
> 10% are bilateral
> 10% are malignant
> 10% are familial

The extra-adrenal form most likely to be malignant is the retroperitoneal (*behind* the peritoneum) form, since cancer sneaks up from *behind*.

PATHOLOGY QUIZ

1. The second most important cause of death in infants is:
   a. Congenital malformations
   b. Accidents
   c. Cancer
   d. Respiratory disease

2. The most important non-accidental cause of death among older children is:
   a. Congenital malformations
   b. Rabies
   c. Cancer
   d. Respiratory disease

3. Which is correct?
   a. Dysplasia precedes metaplasia
   b. Dysplasia precedes cancer
   c. Hodgkin's disease is rarely contiguous in nodal spread
   d. Hodgkin's disease has a tendency for extranodal sites

4. A systolic murmur is heard with:
   a. Aortic stenosis
   b. Mitral stenosis
   c. Aortic insufficiency
   d. Rheumatic heart disease

5. Which is an incorrect association?
   a. Whipple's disease affects the GI of older white men.
   b. Peutz-Jagher affects the GI and lips.
   c. Plummer-Vinson affects the GI of calcium-deficient women.
   d. Pellagra affects the GI and skin.

6. Concerning malignancy, which is true?
   a. CEA levels are markedly depressed in patients with known colon cancer.
   b. Most pheochromocytomas have the capability to metastasize.
   c. Tuberous colon adenomas frequently convert to villous colon adenomas.
   d. Villous colon adenomas more frequently convert to cancer than tuberous adenomas.

7. Which is a classic risk factor for the development of pure cholesterol gall stones?
   a. Lovastatin therapy
   b. Morbidly obese
   c. Male age 25
   d. Celibacy

8. A patient presents with pathologically elevated bilirubin, which is determined to be conjugated. On exploratory surgery of his abdomen, the liver appears dark black.
   a. This patient has indirect hyperbilirubinemia.
   b. This patient has Rotor's disease.
   c. This patient most likely has hemolytic anemia.
   d. This patient may have Dubin-Johnson syndrome.

9. On exploratory surgery of the previous patient, prominent venous dilatation is noted about the esophagus. Which is incorrect?
   a. This patient may be an abuser of alcohol.
   b. This sign supports the diagnosis of Arnold-Chiari syndrome.
   c. Dilation of the hepatic vein may prove beneficial to the patient.
   d. This patient may also have hemorrhoids.

For questions 10-14, match the following diseases with the appropriate risk factors:
   a. Hepatocellular carcinoma
   b. Liver cell adenoma
   c. Primary sclerosing cholangitis
   d. Angiosarcoma
   e. Acute pancreatitis

10. Chronic hepatitis B infection

11. Ulcerative colitis in men

12. Alcohol binge

13. Vinyl chloride

14. Use of oral contraceptives

15. Which is true regarding the genitourinary system?
    a. IgA antibodies are most prominent in the loops of Henle in Berger's disease.
    b. Infertility can be caused by epispadias, since the ejaculate would empty below the cervix.
    c. Nephrotic syndrome should be considered in patients with edematous periorbital skin.
    d. Henoch-Schonlein presents classically with pink loops histologically on kidney biopsy.

16. Which is correctly matched?
    a. Meniere's is increased pressure in the inner ear.
    b. Pterygium is a round lesion on the surface of the eye.
    c. Horner's syndrome causes facial sweating, pupil dilation, and retracted eyelid.
    d. A patient with Hunter's disease usually has eyes which appear to be cloudy.

For questions 17-22, match the following diseases with the most appropriate and specific findings:
    a. Painful, diffusely enlarged thyroid
    b. Centripedal obesity and acne
    c. Adenoma cells on adrenal biopsy
    d. Bilateral unilocular ciliated tumors
    e. Hyperplasia of both adrenals
    f. Absence of thyroid on x-ray
    g. Malodorous
    h. Carcinoma on adrenal biopsy
    i. Unilateral multilocular tumors
    j. None of the above

17. Mucinous ovarian tumor

18. DiGeorge disease

19. PKU

20. Cushing's syndrome

21. Hyperaldosteronism

22. De Quervain's thyroiditis

23. Which is correct?
    a. Nulliparity is correlated with higher risk of breast cancer.
    b. Having many children may protect against cervical cancer.
    c. Early age of first sexual encounter correlates positively with ovarian cancer.
    d. Oral contraceptives increase the risk of ovarian and uterine cancer.

24. Endometrial cancer risk increases with all except:
    a. Obesity
    b. Radiation
    c. Nulliparity
    d. Early menopause

25. Which chromosome is associated with Huntington's disease?
    a. 4
    b. 5
    c. 9
    d. 21

26. A male patient presenting with infertility is found to have "dead" sperm. He is also currently being treated for respiratory disease. Which is also most likely to be found?
    a. Hepatosplenomegaly
    b. A chest x-ray that appears backwards
    c. Family history of cerebrovascular accidents
    d. Chronic cystitis

27. A 3-year-old boy presenting with back pain is found to have cyst-filled kidneys on radiologic study. Which is also most likely to be found?
    a. Hepatosplenomegaly
    b. A chest x-ray that appears backwards
    c. Family history of cerebrovascular accidents
    d. Chronic cystitis

28. A 26-year-old, bed-ridden woman develops DVT's. Which is likely *not* to be a contributing factor?
    a. Prolonged bedrest
    b. Systemic lupus erythematosis
    c. Heparin therapy
    d. Biopsy-proven benign lung mass

PHARMACOLOGY

[Note: Various sources may disagree over the drugs of choice in this section.]

How does botulin act?
Botul-IN keeps it IN. It prevents the release of acetylcholine, thus leading to flaccid paralysis.

How does guanethidine act?
Gua-NE-thidine prevents NE (NorEpinephrine) release.

What do methoxamine and thromboxane do?
They vasoconstrict, as denoted by the OX:

...which is the universal symbol of a constricted vessel lumen.

What are the carbonic anhydrase inhibitors?
The **AMiD**es:

> **A**cetazol**AMIDE**
> **M**ethazol**AMIDE**, and
> **D**ichlorphen**AMIDE**

How do you recognize cholinomimetics?
The suffix "CHOL" as in bethane**CHOL**.

How do you recognize a beta-blocker?
The suffix "OLOL," as in propranOLOL.

What is the shortest-acting beta-blocker?
ESMOLOL IS SMALL (it has the smallest half-life).

Which calcium channel blockers act peripherally (on vessels) and which act more on the heart?
Verapamil and Diltiazem act on the heart, so these don't cause reflex tachycardia and thus put less work on a failing heart. The other CCB's (the "IPINEs") act more in the periphery; this includes the coronaries.

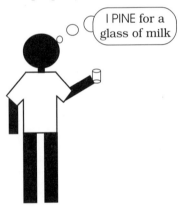

I PINE for a glass of milk

The milk represents CALCIUM channel blockers, held out in the periphery. "IPINE" refers to nifedIPINE, etc.

...But don't leave the milk out in the sun or it'll spoil: IPINE CCB's must be stored in darkness.

What secondary messengers do beta-adrenergics and nitroglycerine act through?

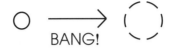

Beta-adrenergic dilates through
c**AMP**
Nitroglycerine dilates through
c**GMP**

What receptors do labetalol bind to?
Labetalol loves it all. It binds to both beta receptors (as "-beta-" and "-alol" imply), as well as alpha-1.

Which alpha-blocker has a longer duration of action, phenoxybenzamine or phentolamine?
The longer word (PB) has the longer duration, as it acts irreversibly.

What are the cardioselective beta-blockers?
A BEAM through your heart:

Atenolol

Betaxolol
Esmolol
Acebutolol
Metoprolol

What is different about lisinopril's effect on the heart?
While most ACE inhibitors cause reflex increase in cardiac output...

> LISINopril may LESSEN cardiac output

What may alert a patient to the toxicity of digitoxin?
A warning light goes on, seen by the patient as a change in color vision.

What are some factors causing male infertility?

CAN'T SWIM

Cimetidine
Alcohol
Nitrofurantoin
Tobacco
Sulfasalazine
Water (hot tubs)
Infection (mumps, TB)
Marijuana

What is the management of an acute M.I.?
THAMES (like the river)

Thrombolytics
Heparin
Aspirin
Morphine (esp. with heart failure)
ECG
Serial enzymes (CK, LDH)

Which muscle relaxants are not cleared by the visceral organs?
SAM has no guts:

> **S**uccinylcholine,
> **A**tracurium, and
> **M**ivacurium are not cleared by the guts.

Which muscle relaxant is cleared mainly by the liver?
Vecuronium is cleared by the li**V**er. The others (aside from SAM) are cleared by the kidneys.

Which general anesthetics will raise intracranial pressure (ICP)?
Ken 'n Hal have big heads:

> **KEN** (**KE**tami**N**e)
> **'n** (**EN**flurane)
> **HAL** (**HAL**othane) have
> big heads *(increase ICP)*

Other general anesthetics lower ICP.

What is etomidate for?
Etomidate is a general anesthetic for patients with heart disease.

> Little Tommy has a bad heart.

TOMmy is e**TOM**idate. He's *little*; likewise, etomidate is only for *short* use, because of adrenocortical depression.

What are three drugs causing thrombocytopenia?
THrombo**C**yto**P**enia:

> **TH**iazides
> **S**ulfas *(C and S sound the same)*
> **P**enicillin

What are the NSAID's, aside from aspirin?
The "PRO" drugs: ibu**PRO**fen, keto**PRO**fen, na**PRO**xen. All have the same efficacy.

How is rheumatoid arthritis treated?
1. Aspirin. If this fails, try...
2. NSAID's. If nothing works, try...
3. MALARIA, GOLD, and CANCER

> MALARIA (chloroquine)
> GOLD (auro drugs)
> CANCER (methotrexate,
>   cyclophosphamide)

How do you treat chronic gout?
Try to **SAP** the uric acid out of him (via increasing its excretion).

> **S**ulfinpyrazole
> **A**llopurinol
> **P**robenecid

How do you treat acute gout?
Never give aspirin or allopurinol to a man with acute gout. You can, however, give:
1. NSAID's
2. Colchicine

What are the effects of morphine?
Morphine shuts out the world and shuts down the body:

1. Decreases pain perception
2. Increases sleep
3. Decreases respiration
4. Constricts the pupils
5. Decreases GI motility
6. Causes urinary retention

In addition, morphine causes emesis and convulsions. It is effective, however, as an antitussive.

Reliable symptoms in the emergency room of morphine toxicity are the three C's:

> **C**onstricted pupils
> **C**onstipation
> **C**onvulsion

What combination of abused substances can cause a fatal withdrawal?
Alcohol and **B**arbiturates.

What are the opioids?
In decreasing potency:

> Fentanyl
> Heroin
> Methadone
> — Morphine —
> Meperidine
> Codeine
> Propoxyphene

Which of these narcotics causes mydriasis?
MEPERidine. (Sing to tune of "Jeepers Creepers")...

MEEPERS creepers
Where'd you get them peepers?
MEEPERS creepers
Where'd you get those *eyes?*

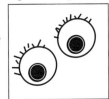

(If you're not familiar with the song, nevermind.)

How may a person on PCP appear?
The four C's of PCP...

> **C**ombative
> **C**atatonic
> **C**onvulsing
> **C**omatose

Is loperamide an abused substance?
LOperamide has LOW abuse potential.

Does marijuana have any medicinal value?
To quote Dylan, "Everybody must get stoned." He was, of course, referring to the variety of people who would benefit from THC therapy:

1. Children with ASTHMA (marijuana is a bronchodilator)
2. Elderly patients with GLAUCOMA (marijuana decreases intraocular pressure)
3. Everyone in-between on CANCER CHEMOTHERAPY (marijuana is an anti-emetic)

Remember to look in the eyes of all stuporous patients. Those on marijuana will have bloodshot eyes. Those on PCP will have vertical and horizontal nystagmus. Cocaine dilates. Morphine constricts.

Why is MDMA ("XTC," "Adam") so bad for you?
MDMA acts like a MaDMAn; it kills the serotonin-containing neurons.

What are the benzodiazepines?
The "PAM" drugs (flurazepam, diazepam, lorazepam, and temazepam). PAM is a woman who has trouble sleeping. Triazolam is also a benzo, but has a much shorter half-life than the PAMs.

Don't be confused by chlorDIAZEpoxide. It's a benzoDIAZEpine as well.

What are the barbiturates?
The "AL" drugs (phenobarbital, pentobarbital, and thiopental). AL is a man addicted to barbs.

What is chloral hydrate?
Looking at all the pretty CORAL under the sea is relaxing. CHLORAL hydrate also puts you to sleep.

What is buspirone?
BUSpirone is used safely by the nervous BUS driver; it's an anxiolytic which won't cause sedation. It is the alternative to benzos. As with other main alternatives, it acts via serotonin *(see pages 117 and 119)*.

Antiepileptic	Indication
Phenobarbital	Febrile seizures
Diazepam	Opisthotonic seizure and status epilepticus; Barbiturate withdrawal
Phenytoin	Partial and tonic-clonic seizures
Carbamazepine	Partial and tonic-clonic seizures
Valproic acid	Absence seizures
Ethosuximide	Absence seizures

What are the side effects of phenytoin?
When on PHENYtoin you become FUNNY-looking. You can get hirsutism and gingival hyperplasia.

What are the side effects of carbamazepine?
CArbAmAzepine causes **A**plastic **A**nemia and **A**granulocytosis.

As a general rule, most antipsychotics are low-potency except FLUPHENAZINE and HALOPERIDOL:

	Mechanism	Side Effects
Low potency	blocks alpha, muscarinic, & histaminic receptors	hypotension, blurred vision, urinary retention, dry mouth
High potency	blocks dopamine receptor	Parkinsonian (EPS[*])
Clozapine	blocks serotonin	hypersalivation, fatal agranulocytosis

[*]EPS = Extra Pyramidal Side effects

How does clozapine act?
Clozapine is the alternative antipsychotic. Like buspirone, the alternative anxiolytic, it acts on serotonin. Like the ad says, "They used to put you in the CLOSet... now they put you on CLOZapine."

Which antipsychotic is good for hiccups?
Chlorpromazine, the prototypical antipsychotic.

Which antipsychotic is not an antiemetic?
ThioRIDazine. You vomit and get RID of your lunch.

Here is a way to organize the TriCyclic Antidepressants (TCAs):
There are two types, the secondary (2°) and the tertiary (3°) amines. The 2° amines operate via norepinephrine (NE), while the 3° amines act via serotonin (5HT). Associate **3°** with **5HT**...

2°	3°
NE	**5HT**

NE can be rewritten as ND (standing for **N**ortriptyline and **D**esipramine), while HT looks like AI (**A**mitriptyline and **I**mipramine) if you squint really hard:

2°	3°
NE	5HT
ND	AI

What are the other (2nd and 3rd generation) popular antidepressants?

FAT

> **F**luoxetine (Prozac)
> **A**moxapine
> **T**razodone

Maprotiline is also in this group, though not as popular.

How does Prozac work?
It is the main alternative to the traditional antidepressants. It thus acts via serotonin (refer to buspirone and clozapine as well).

What is the important side effect of amoxapine?
a**MOX**apine **MOCKS** a neuroleptic. Hence, it has extrapyramidal side effects.

Also note that trazodone's important side effect is priapism.

What are MAOI's?
They are antidepressants with a "YL" in the name, like tranYLcypromine and phenYLzine.

Coverage of Antibiotics:

GRAM POSITIVE (the cins):
      bacitraCIN
      erythromyCIN
      vancomyCIN
      clindamyCIN
      also... 1st and 2nd generation PENICILLINS

GRAM NEGATIVE (memorize these):
      polymyxin
      aminoglycosides (see pages 121 and 122)
      aztreonam
      4th generation penicillins

BROAD SPECTRUM:
      everything else

What drug increases the bioavailability of penicillin by decreasing its excretion?
Probenecid, the same drug that *increases* the excretion of uric acid in gout patients.

What are the penicillin derivatives, in order of generation?

"**GiVe Me A T**aste of **Pie**"

1st generation:	pen **G** and **V** (GiVe)
2nd generation:	**Me**thicillin (Me), also Nafcillin
3rd generation:	**A**mpicillin and Amoxicillin (A)
4th generation:	**T**icarcillin (Taste of)
5th generation:	**Pi**peracillin (Pie)

What are the three classes of cephalosporins used for?

1st generation	prophylaxis before "dirty" (GI) surgery	$\oplus > \ominus$
2nd generation	beta-lactamase *H. influenzae*	$\oplus = \ominus$
3rd generation	meningitis	$\oplus < \ominus$

Plus/minus signs refer to efficacy in treating gram positive versus negative infections. The generations go from positive to negative.

What antibiotics block translation?

Think of **STCEP** (looks like STREP):

- **S**treptomycin binds to the 30S before any translation can occur. Hence, a 30S-50S complex cannot form.

- **T**etracycline allows the complex to form, but sits in the A site and doesn't let any more translocation occur.

- **C**hloramphenicol (and Cycloheximide) let the A site become occupied, but then prevent peptidyl transferase from binding.

- **E**rythromycin lets peptidyl transferase come in and bind, but then prevents translocation from proceeding.

- **P**uromycin lets translation proceed until it occupies the A site and then binds to the growing chain, thus stopping translation.

Note that cycloheximide acts in eukaryotes, so it isn't popular. Also note that clindaMYCIN and erythroMYCIN show cross-resistance.

What organisms do aminoglycosides cover?
aMINOglycoSIDES are CIDAL (deadly) to a MINUS (gram negative).

What are the major side effects of aminoglycosides and which drugs have them?

All are considered nephrotoxic. The ototoxic aminoglycosides are subdivided into those that diminish hearing, and those that alter balance:

HEARING (**KAN'T** hear)	BALANCE (**S**ome **G**et **T**ipsy)
Kanamycin	**S**treptomycin
Amikacin	**G**entamicin
Neomycin	**T**obramycin
Tobramycin	

This mnemonic appears courtesy of Dr. Donald McMillan.

What are the sulfa drugs for?

- Sodium sulFACEtamide is for the FACE (topical use only); the short-acting sulfa is for UTI's

- SulFAMEthoxazole with trimethoprim (Bactrim) for *P. carinii* in AIDS patients

- SulFADoxine with pyrimethamine for *P. falciparum* in malaria patients
  ...because in the USA, AIDS is FAMous while malaria is merely a FAD.

Note: Don't confuse pyrazinamide for TB with pyriMethamine for Malaria.

What is the treatment of leprosy?
DR. Leper

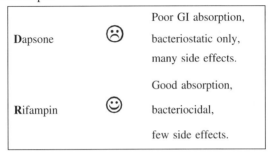

| **D**apsone | ☹ | Poor GI absorption, bacteriostatic only, many side effects. |
| **R**ifampin | ☺ | Good absorption, bacteriocidal, few side effects. |

See the Microbiology chapter (p. 147) for treatment of TB.

What are the drugs of choice in tapeworm, roundworm, and fluke infections?
- TAPEWORMS need NICLOSAMIDE
- ROUNDWORMS need MEBENDAZOLE (BENDing something makes it ROUND)
- FLUKES need PRAZIQUANTAL

The drug praziquantal breaks a few rules, so we call it CRAZY PRAZI...

1. The exception to tapeworms is *T. solium* which needs PRAZIquantal; solium means sun, which is bright. But Crazy Prazi is not terribly bright.
2. The flukes are fluky and need Crazy Prazi also.
3. The drugs listed above act by inhibiting glucose uptake, except Crazy Prazi which increases calcium permeability.

*Also note that there are a few exceptions among the roundworms: use THIAbendazole for strongyloides, *T. spiralis*, and *A. braziliense*.

What is the drug for herpetic encephalitis?
When you're PSYCHO you need aCYCLOvir (sort of sound alike). Vidarabine also works.

What is the drug for CMV retinitis?
Gancyclovir for CMV (G and C look alike).

What is the drug for herpetic keratoconjunctivitis?
Iododeoxyuridine for **EYE** (I) infections.

Note: Most other herpetic infections use acyclovir.

What is the drug for RSV?
Ribavirin is for **R**SV.

What is the drug for influenza A?
Amantad**IN**e is for **IN**fluenz**A**

What are the drugs used for nonviral STD's?
- Sy**P**hilis is treated with **P**enicillin
- Gono**C**occus is treated with **C**eftriaxone
- Chlamy**D**ia is treated with **D**oxycycline

What are the commonly seen tick-borne vectors and their treatments?

You're reading a mystery novel and want to know the murderer. You can either...

Try **G**uessing or **R**ead **T**he **L**ast **P**age

> **T**ularemia treated with **G**entamicin;
> **R**ickettsia treated with **T**etracycline;
> **L**yme disease treated with **P**enicillin.

What are cosyntropin and protirelin analogs of?

Bill COSBY used to ACT, but since he RETIRED he plays the TRACKS.

COSb**Y** is **COSY**ntropin	*cosyntropin is an*
ACT is **ACT**H	*analogue of ACTH*
re**TIRE**d is pro**TIRE**lin	*protirelin is an*
TRACKS is **TR**H	*analogue of TRH*

What is gonadorelin used for?

Like the name implies, it's an analogue of GONADOtropin RELeasINg hormone, used for hypogonadism.

What is octreotide used for?

In the James Bond film *OCTopussy*, Bond had to fight Jaws. The actor who played Jaws has acromegaly. Hence, OCTreotide is used to lower GH in patients with acromegaly.

---

*What are desmo*pressin *and l*pressin*?*
Two forms of vaso*pressin*. These PRESS on the vessels and cause constriction.

What form is estradiol given in?
As an intra-muscular OIL, not orally... estradIOL is estradOIL.

What is tamoxifen used for?
It can be used for breast cancer if the cancer has estrogen receptors. Tammy is a woman with breast cancer, so TAMoxiFEN is TAMmy's FriENd.

What is danazol used for?
Endometriosis and fibrocystic disease. DANA is a woman with both of these, so DANAZOL gets it ALL.

How is medroxyprogesterone given?
The ME of MEdroxyprogesterone means I AM, which sounds like I.M. Hence, it can be given I.M. (intramuscularly).

What is RU486?
It's an antiprogesterone known as mifepristone, a controversial abortifacient. MIFepriSTONE has people MIFFED and throwing STONEs. RU486 or against it?

What is gossypol?
What's the GOSSIP ALL about? It's about GOSSYPOL, the male contraceptive.

What does fludrocortisol do?
FLUDrocortisol stops the FLOOD. It stops polyuria by stimulating salt water retention.

What causes constipation, aluminum hydroxide or magnesium hydroxide?
Of these two antacids, ALUMINUM hydroxide causes constipation while magnesium hydroxide causes diarrhea. If you swallow an aluminum can, it'll get stuck in your GI and lead to constipation.

Note: Magnesium SULFATE is not an antacid, it's a saline cathartic (stimulates bowel movement).

How does omeprazole act?
By inhibiting the gastric mucosal hydrogen-potassium ATPase...

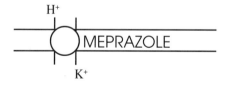

How does sucralfate help GI ulcers?
suCRAlfate covers the CRAter by forming an epithelial lining.

How does misoprostol act?
MisoPROSTol is a PROSTaglandin analogue, which protects the mucosa.

How do H₂ blockers act?
They inhibit acid release in the stomach, thus preventing heartburn after meals. Hence, as the suffix "IDINE" (e.g., cimetIDINE) implies, they let you DINE. A person with gastroesophageal reflux would say, "Before I DINE, I take my H₂ blockers."

What does metoclopramide do?
META makes you MOTILE. It stimulates the gut.

What do laxatives do?
LAXatives reLAX the stool and thus ease defecation.

Which is cycle-specific, azothioprine or cyclophosphamide?
Azothioprine is cycle-specific. CYCLOphosphamide is PSYCHO, and kills regardless of cycle phase (it's not cycle-specific).

What are the side effects of some chemotherapeutic agents?

Agent	Side Effect(s)
Cyclophosphamide	hemorrhagic Cystitis
Methotrexate	Me+ho+reXa+e has some nasty spikes, so swallowing it causes hemorrhagic enteritis
Vincristine/ Vinblastine	Peripheral neuropathy (the nerves are the first to go when you abuse VIN [French for wine])
DaunoRUBicin/ DoxoRUBicin	Cardiotoxicity (RUBies are red, like a heart)
Bleomycin	Pulmonary fibrosis (BLEO makes it hard to BLOW)
ciSPLATin	Same as AMINOglycocides (nephro and ototoxicity): a man jumped off a building and went SPLAT, because it's A-MEAN-OL' world

What DNA base is most susceptible to alkylation?
Guanine **G**ets it

What are the preferred therapies for colon and rectal cancers?
Colon cancer gets **C**hemo, while **R**ectal cancer gets **R**adiation.

What are signs of organophosphate toxicity?

SLUM
Salivation
Lacrimation
Urination
Miosis

What organ does lead toxicity spare?
Lead affects many organs but **L**eaves the **L**iver a**L**one.

What human protein helps prevent cadmium toxicity?
Metallothionein...
- CADMIUM sounds like the hollow chocolate CADBURY bunny, which is EMPTY inside.
- EMPTY = MT = MetalloThionein.

No drugs chelate cadmium.

Which is cleared by dimercaprol, organic or inorganic mercury?
d**I**-**MERC**aprol clears **I**norganic **MERC**ury, not organic. It also clears other metals, but not lead.

What drug clears lead?
Ca-EDTA. Don't confuse Calcium-EDTA (a lead chelator) with EDTA (a calcium chelator). Don't be misLEAD!

What does methemoglobin do to iron?
Converts it from the normal Fe^{+2} to Fe^{+3}. *(See p. 70.)*

What does deferoxamine do?
DEFEROXamine DETOXes FEROX. You treat iron overload with it.

Drugs of Choice:

Symptom	Drug
Neuromuscular blockade reversal	Neostigmine
Myasthenia gravis diagnosis	Edrophonium
Myasthenia gravis therapy	Pyridostigmine
Antimuscarinic toxicity	Physostigmine
Organophosphate toxicity	Atropine and Pralidoxime
To keep ductus arteriosus patent	PGE_2
To close a patent ductus	Indomethacin

Symptom	Drug
Acute gout	Indomethacin
Hypertensive crisis	Nitroprusside
High triglycerides	Gemfibrozil
Heparin toxicity	Protamine
Ongoing coronary occlusion	Streptokinase (not heparin)
Chronic diabetes insipidus	Desmopressin
Thyroid replacement	Levothyroxine
Paget's disease of bone	Calcitonin/Etidronate
Cortisol replacement	Hydrocortisone
Acute inflammation (systemic)	Dexamethasone
Chronic inflammation (systemic)	Prednisone
Rheumatoid arthritis	Aspirin
Opioid overdose	Naloxone / naltrexone
Opioid detoxification	Methadone
C. difficile	Vancomycin
Legionnaire's disease	Erythromycin
Anaerobes	Clindamycin

PHARMACOLOGY QUIZ

1. Which is true?
   a. The toxin that causes botulism causes massive release of acetylcholine
   b. Thromboxane is an endogenously produced vasodilator
   c. Esmolol is a beta-blocker with a short half-life
   d. Phentolamine is an irreversibly binding alpha-blocker

2. Which is not considered a cardioselective beta-blocker?
   a. Esmolol
   b. Propranolol
   c. Atenolol
   d. Metoprolol

3. Which is a carbonic anhydrase inhibitor?
   a. Dichlorphenamide
   b. Spironolactone
   c. Mannitol
   d. Furosemide

4. Which is correct?
   a. Nifedipine is associated with reflex tachycardia
   b. Diltiazem is a centrally acting ACE inhibitor
   c. Verapamil is ineffective if exposed to light
   d. Lisinopril is a centrally acting calcium channel blocker

5. Of the following muscle relaxants, which is not cleared by the liver or kidneys?
   a. Vecuronium
   b. Doxacurium
   c. d-Tubocurarine
   d. Succinylcholine

6. Which anesthetic does not raise intracranial pressure?
   a. Halothane
   b. Etomidate
   c. Ketamine
   d. Enflurane

7. Choose the incorrect association:
   a. Aspirin for rheumatoid arthritis
   b. NSAIDs for acute gout
   c. Aspirin for acute gout
   d. NSAIDs for rheumatoid arthritis

8. Which of the following is not a likely cause of male infertility?
   a. Beer
   b. Cigarettes
   c. Marijuana
   d. Coffee

9. A 58-year-old man with a known history of M.I. presents with chest pain radiating to his left arm, profuse sweating, and bibasilar lung crackles. His ECG shows signs of new myocardial injury, and his CK-MB fraction is elevated. Which drug would not reduce this patient's mortality risk?
    a. Phenobarbital
    b. Aspirin
    c. Morphine
    d. Streptokinase

10. Which is a common side effect of morphine?
    a. Diarrhea
    b. Miosis
    c. Tachypnea
    d. Urinary incontinence

11. Which drug may cause death upon abrupt discontinuation of chronic use?
    a. Beer
    b. Cocaine
    c. Valium (diazepam)
    d. Heroin

12. Which opioid is associated with mydriasis?
    a. Heroin
    b. Codeine
    c. Meperidine
    d. Methadone

13. A 16-year-old boy presents in a coma after having attempted several illicit drugs at once. He is breathing slowly, and ocular examination reveals markedly injected (bloodshot) eyes in vertical nystagmus. His pupils do not dilate. Which of the following drugs should you least consider to be a contributing cause of his condition?
    a. Marijuana
    b. PCP
    c. Cocaine
    d. Heroin

14. Which medication is least likely to sedate?
    a. Chloral hydrate
    b. Buspirone
    c. Lorazepam
    d. Thiopental

15. Which is a correct drug of choice for seizures?
    a. Valproic acid for status epilepticus
    b. Diazepam for absence seizures
    c. Phenytoin for febrile seizures
    d. Ethosuxamide for absence seizures

16. Which antiepileptic causes gingival hyperplasia and hirsutism?
    a. Phenytoin
    b. Diazepam
    c. Valproic acid
    d. Carbamazepine

17. Which medication does not act via serotonin?
    a. Clozapine
    b. Clonidine
    c. Fluoxetine (Prozac)
    d. Buspirone

18. Which is true?
    a. Thioridazine may be used as an effective antiemetic
    b. Fluoxetine (Prozac) is a commonly prescribed antipsychotic
    c. A major disadvantage to amoxapine is its extrapyramidal side effects
    d. Desipramine is a tertiary amine TCA

For questions 19-25, match each of the following antibiotics with its appropriate coverage:
    a. Primarily gram positive organisms
    b. Primarily gram negative organisms
    c. Broad spectrum

19. Chloramphenicol

20. Third-generation cephalosporins

21. Erythromycin

22. Aminoglycosides

23. First-generation penicillins

24. Ticarcillin

25. Ampicillin

26. Which is incorrectly matched?
    a. Sodium sulfacetamide is for topical use only
    b. Bactrim (sulfamethoxazole and trimethoprim) is used for *P. carinii* infections
    c. Sulfadoxine and pyrimethamine are used for malarial infections
    d. Sulfamethoxazole and pyrimethamine are used for tuberculosis infections

27. Which is correct?
    a. Dapsone is an effective drug for leprosy as it is bacteriocidal
    b. Rifampin is an effective drug for TB but is only bacteriostatic
    c. Dapsone is an effective drug for TB but is poorly absorbed through the GI
    d. Rifampin is an effective drug for leprosy as it has good GI absorption

28. The most effective medication for CMV retinitis is:
    a. Gancyclovir
    b. Acyclovir
    c. Ribavirin
    d. Amantadine

29. The most effective medication for RSV is:
    a. Gancyclovir
    b. Acyclovir
    c. Ribavirin
    d. Amantadine

Questions 30-34: Match each of the following medications with its appropriate coverage:
   a. Penicillin
   b. Tetracycline or doxycycline
   c. Ceftriaxone
   d. Gentamicin

30. Infant with Lyme disease

31. Syphilis

32. Tularemia

33. Rocky Mountain Spotted Fever

34. Chlamydia

35. Which is correct?
   a. Estradiol is a popular ingredient in oral contraceptives
   b. Medroxyprogesterone is only found in oral contraceptives
   c. Mifepristone (RU486) inhibits implantation by the conceptus
   d. Gossypol acts mainly by its effects on the menstrual cycle

36. Which is matched correctly?
   a. Omeprazole acts by creating a mucosal lining
   b. Metoclopramide causes constipation
   c. Ranitidine acts by inhibiting the hydrogen-potassium ATPase
   d. Aluminum hydroxide causes constipation

37. Which drug is incorrectly matched with its side effect?
    a. Cyclophosphamide causes pulmonary fibrosis
    b. Doxorubicin causes cardiac disease
    c. Cisplatin causes nephrotoxicity and ototoxicity
    d. Vincristine causes neuropathy

38. A 42-year-old farmer presents to the E.R. with complaints of tearing and drooling. On exam his pupils are fixed and miotic, and he smells of urine. This patient most likely:
    a. Also harvests marijuana, and has recently burned a large crop to avoid detection
    b. Has had a significant cutaneous exposure to insecticide
    c. Was up with the boys drinking homemade moonshine made from radiator fluid
    d. Has recently eaten home-canned fruits contaminated with *C. botulinum*

39. Which is correct?
    a. Lead causes significant hepatotoxicity
    b. Lead toxicity is treated with administration of metallothionein
    c. Dimercaprol is used in the treatment of organic mercury toxicity
    d. Deferoxamine is useful in treating significant iron supplement overdose

MICROBIOLOGY AND IMMUNOLOGY

What infections do a deficiency in B cells predispose one to?
B cell deficiency allows more **B**acterial infections. T cell deficiency allows other forms of infection.

How are germinal centers arranged in lymph tissue?
The central areas make B cells, while tissue between the centers makes T cells:

What is agammaglobulinemia of Bruton?
Bruton means only *BRUTES* (men) get it due to the X-linked inheritance, and **B** cells are deficient.

What are the hypersensitivity reactions?
Type one: IMMEDIATE (IgE mediated, anaphylactic)
Type two: AUTOIMMUNE (cytotoxic)
Type three: COMPLEX deposition
Type four: DELAYED (T cell mediated)

> **I'm A Complex Dude**
> I'm = Immediate
> A = Autoimmune
> Complex = Complex deposition
> Dude = Delayed

Which is made first: IgD or IgM?
B cells present IgM first, then IgD; the B cell must have an MD to be competent (just like doctors). Similarly, these B cells first release M, then G antibodies upon primary exposure.

What causes mast cell degranulation, cGMP or cAMP?
When you sit in an Andy Gump (GMP), you release your contents (for a mast cell, degranulate):

> increasing cGMP stimulates degranulation
> increasing cAMP inhibits degranulation

Note: Andy Gump is a popular outhouse.

Which Major Histocompatibility Complexes are on T cells?

MHC I associates with T_8 } $1 \times 8 = 2 \times 4$
MHC II associates with T_4

- In addition, T_C (for cytotoxic T cells) looks like T_ε (which resembles T_8 [CD8]).
- T_h (for helper T cells) resembles T_μ which looks like T_4 (CD4).

What do the subunits of diphtheria toxin do?

A Attacks the cell;
B Binds the cell surface:

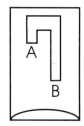

An experimentor adds human B and T cells to sheep RBCs and sees rosettes. What is the human cell that caused this?
The T cell.

When you
see this:

You should
think this:

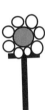

What antibody moves across the placenta?
Ig**G** **G**oes.

What antibodies contain a J chain?
JAM: **J** is in Ig**A** and **M**

What components aid in anaphylaxis?
A is for *A*naphylaxis (C3*a*, 4*a*, and 5*a*). (C3b is involved in opsonization).

Do the bacterial cell wall peptides bind to NAM or NAG?

NAG nags them, so they hang with NAM.

What bacteria possess teichoic acid, pili, and spores?

Gram **+** possess **+**eichoic acid.

Gram **—** possess P | L |.

Gram **P**ositive also have s**P**ores.

(Note: Refer to pharmacology section for antibiotics.)

Here's how to organize the Gram-stainable pathogenic bacteria:

		Rods	
	Cocci	*Aerobes*	*Anaerobes*
Gram Positive	StaPh StreP	Diphtheria Listeria	Actinomyces Bacillus Clostridium
Gram Negative	Neisseria	*Everything else*	

Don't confuse Bacillus (gram *positive* anaerobic rod) with Bacteroides (gram *negative* anaerobic rod). *Nocardia* is a group of aerobic rods that may be acid fast or stain positive.

What are the proteins of staph and strep?
stAPH has proteins A-F (stA-F aureus), while strep
has protein M.

Does Staph Scalded Skin Syndrome cause scars?
No, **SSSS** is **S**an**S** **S**car**S**.

Which is catalase positive, staph or strep?
Staph is CATalase positive; strep is not. Staph means
grape-like, so think of a CAT eating grapes.

---

*What alpha-hemolytic streps cause GREEN hemolysis
on blood agar?*
- Verde is Spanish for green. Hence, *Strep
  VIRIDans* makes green colonies.
- *Strep pneumoniae* produces green sputum.

Who mostly gets strep A versus B?
- A is for Adults
- B is for Babies

What are the "grey bugs"?
Two organisms grow out grey colonies. *C.
diphtheriae* is plated on tellurite, and *Listeria* on
blood agar. These also happen to be the only two
pathogenic gram positive aerobic rods.

What do you plate C. diphtheriae *on? (No looking!)*
Just remember the old radio ad:
"Does pharyngeal pseudomembrane have your patients
unable to speak?
    "Then TELLURITE will TELL-YOU-RIGHT."

What are the important pathogenic anaerobes?

A B C: **A**ctinomyces
              Bacteroides
              Clostridium

How do Bacteroides and Clostridium stain?
Like the borderline grade of C+/B-

> Clostridium stains positive (C plus)
> Bacteroides stains negative (B minus)

---

*These three groups are often confused, and can be
sorted as follows:*

Bacteroides	Clostridium	Bacillus
anaerobes	anaerobes	aerobes
(NO to O_2)	*(NO to O_2)*	
NO spores	spores	spores
gram Negative	gram positive	gram positive
(very negative bugs)	(fairly positive bugs)	(very positive bugs)

Are actinomyces fungi?
No, actinomyces are just actin' like myces (fungi);
they're really gram positive bacteria.

Is Bacteroides fragilis *fragile?*

No. In fact, the organism has a capsule, so it's far from fragile. It is the GI mucosa that is fragile; this organism is only pathogenic once it gets past a tear in the fragile GI mucosa.

What are the anti-TB drugs of choice (as of 1993)?

RIPE

> **R**ifampin
> **I**soniazid
> **P**yrazinamide
> **E**thambutol

What are some unique attributes of these TB drugs?

A B C:

Atypical mycobacteria susceptible
B$_6$ supplements needed
CNS susceptible to infection

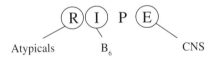

Atypicals   B$_6$ CNS

What is the action of tetracycline (previously used for TB)?

tetracycline blocks **t**RNA.

What about rifampin?

Rifampin inhibits **R**NA synthesis. It also colors body fluids **R**ed.

What is the action of isoniazid?
Isoniazid inhibits mYcolic acid synthesis (different letter, but close enough).

How does Asteroides *stain?*
ASTeroides is Acid-faST.

How is Legionnaire's disease spread?
Legionnaire's is in the air, not person to person.

What assay can diagnose Mycoplasma pneumoniae*?*
The COLD agglutinin test. *Mycoplasma* has no coat, so it's COLD.

What does a Mycoplasma *colony look like?*
Like a fried egg. And like fried eggs, *Mycoplasma* is infamous for its cholesterol.

What are eschars?
Eschars can be seen in anthrax. They are big black spots on the skin, contracted from cows, which also have big black spots on their skin.

What organisms should be suspected in meningitis?
The encapsulated ones:
*   *Strep pneumoniae*
*   *Neisseria meningitidis*
*   *Haemophilus influenzae*
*   *Cryptococcus neoformans*

Does Neisseria have oxidase?
NO, as in: yes, **N**eisseria has **O**xidase.

What organism causes opthalmia neonatorium?
GONorrhea

> **G**onorrhea causes
> **O**pthalmia
> **N**eonatorium

How do you identify the two pathogenic Neisseria organisms by sugar fermentation?

> *N. **G**onorrhoeae* ferments **G**lucose
> *N. **M**enin**G**itidis* ferments **M**altose and **G**lucose

---

How do Campylobacter *and cholera look microscopically?*
Campy and **C**holera appear **C**-shaped.

Which one is painful?
CAMPY is CRAMPY. Cholera is not.

Is Salmonella *motile?*
Yes, just like salmon.

How is salmonella food poisoning acquired?
Salmonella bacteria live in animals (such as
SALMON); you need to eat a whole lotta salmon to
get sick, so the innoculation dose must be high.

Shigella, on the other hand, is only in humans and
requires a low dose for disease to occur (i.e., its
potency is high).

Food Poisonings:

Culprit	Incu- bation	Presentation
Staph aureus	1-8 hrs	N and V; maybe diarrhea
C. perfringens	8-16 hrs	Diarrhea and cramps lasting <24 hrs
B. cereus	(depends)	Looks like either of the above
Salmonella	6-48 hrs.	First N and V, then diarrhea, fever and cramps; maybe blood in stool
Shigella	1-4 days	Fever, cramps, diarrhea; maybe blood in stool
V. cholera		Rice water stool without fever or pain; raw seafood eaten
Campy. jejuni		Bloody diarrhea, fever, and pain without N and V; chicken eaten
E. coli		Returning from travel

How is typhoid fever transmitted?
Via the 5 F's:
> Food, Fingers, Feces, Fomites, and Flies

What does botulin do?
BotulIN keeps it IN (prevents acetylcholine release from nerves).

What organisms penetrate the bowel mucosa?

CS YEAST:

Campylobacter jejuni
Salmonella
Yersinia pestis
E. Coli (certain forms)
Aeromonas
Shigella

What are the symptoms of Reiter's syndrome?
The three C's...

> Chlamydia infection recently
> Calf arthritis (i.e., painful knees and ankles)
> Conjunctivitis

What cause chancres and chancroids?
- Chancres are caused by syphilis and are PAINLESS.
- Chancroids, like hemorrhoids, are PAINFUL and are caused by *Haemophilus DUCREYI* (you DO-CRY, due to the pain).

Here are the rules and exceptions of the Rickettsiae:

- All are obligate intracellular except *R. quintana* (trench fever)
- All are transmitted by bug bite except *C. burnetti* (Q fever)
- All are zoonotic except *R. prowazekii* (epidemic typhus)
- The typical finding is a rash except Q fever (lungs and liver)

Where does the Rocky Mountain Spotted Fever rash appear?

ROCKY Mountain fever starts on the hands, like you've been throwing ROCKS. This is in contrast to the epidemic typhus, which starts on the trunk.

Rashes:

Rash	Presentation
Rocky Mountain Spotted Fever	Hands, then trunk
Epidemic typhus and Varicella (chicken pox)	Trunk, then hands
Smallpox and Rubella	Head, then trunk
Measles	Oral mucosa, then head, then trunk
Coxsackie A	Hands and feet only
Lyme disease	Expanding ring around bite, then migrating

How does Sporothrix shenkii look microscopically?
Sporothrix is commonly transmitted by the thorn of a rose. Hence, it looks like a flower microscopically.

Where do you get coccidioidomycosis, histoplasmosis, and blastomycosis?
Coccidio is gotten in **C**alifornia
HIstoplasmosis is gotten in **OHI**o.
Blastomycosis is gotten from **B**eavers

How does Tinea versicolor *present?*
- Clinically, *Tinea versicolor* is *versatile* in *color*. It may cause a patch that is white or black.
- Microscopically, it is also *versatile*. It presents as both yeast and hyphae.

What are the symptoms of measles?
The three C's...

Cough
Coryza
Conjunctivitis

***Blastomyces** is a **B**road-**B**ased **B**udding yeast:*

What viruses cause retinitis and leukoplakia in AIDS patients?
CMV causes retinitis so you can't **C** (see).
EBV causes leukoplakia so you can't **E**at.

How is CMV transmitted?
CMV is the abbreviation of "**SEE** it **MoVe**." That's because it moves everywhere (blood, intercourse, mom's milk, placenta).

What are the LIVE vaccines?

MR. SPAMY:

> **M**easles
> **R**ubella
>
> **S**mall pox
> **P**olio *(Sabin)*
> **A**denovirus
> **M**umps
> **Y**ellow virus

What are the KILLED vaccines?

R.I.P. *(as in, "Rest in Peace")*

> **R**abies
> **I**nfluenza
> **P**olio *(Salk)*

- Hepatitis B vaccine is also killed.
- Sal**K** is **K**illed. Sabine is live.

> VarioLA causes smaLL pox
> VaCcinia causes Cow pox

What smear diagnoses herpes simplex?
The Tzanck smear... "Tzancks a lot for the herpes!"

How are the hepatitis viruses transmitted?
- You **EA**t heps **E** and **A**.
- Hep B is like AIDS.
- Hep C is the most common form in blood transfusions.
- Hep **D** is **D**efective and relies on hep B.

What are the ingredients of Reye's disease?
ABC:
- **A**spirin
- influenza **B**
- **C**hicken pox

What kind of virus causes rubella?
A togavirus. The guys from Animal House wore *togas* and were *rebels* (they got rebella).

How does rabies affect bats and rabbits?

> BATS don't get BATTY, and
> RABBITS don't get RABID

That is, bats don't appear rabid but do transmit the disease; rabbits don't transmit the disease.

What viruses does the PICORNA group contain?
The RHINOvirus and the ENTEROvirus:

PI (C) ORN

don't PIC your NOSE   eat CORN
(nose = rhino)   (eating = entero)

How do you detect rotavirus infection?
STOOL sample:

> A ROTAting STOOL

What do Coxsackieviruses A and B cause?

A causes Herpangina

B causes Pleurodynia

Note: Herpangina is not angina; and Pleurodynia includes chest pain that may be confused with angina.

Where do the two parasitic forms of Toxoplasma gondii *reside in man?*
The **T**achyzoite lives in the **T**ummy;
The **B**radyzoite lives in the **B**rain

How does Chaga's disease (Trypanosoma cruzi) *affect the esophagus?*
CHAgAS causes a**CHAlAS**ia

What do Diphyllobothrium latum *eggs look like?*
They look like eggs cracked open on top...
"I'm surprised DE FELLA BOTHERED TO LAY
DEM," since they're defective (operculated).

What animals carry T. solium *and* T. saginatum?
- The smaller animal (pig) carries the smaller word (*solium*).
- The larger animal (cow) carries the larger word (*saginatum*)

How does fish tapeworm disturb the patient's nutritional status?
FISH tapeworm causes B12 de-FISH-ency.

What organ does Acanthamoeba *infect?*
Acanthamoeba sounds like *I-can't-rememba*, since it infects the brain. It enters via skin cuts.

How does one contract Naegleria fowleri?
It is like a *fowl* that flies up your nose and also infects the brain.

How do you identify an S. mansoni *egg?*
It has a knife, like Charles Manson:

Here are the trematodes:

Infected SNAIL sheds parasite			
↓	↓	↓	↓
HUMAN eats infected LETTUCE	HUMAN eats CRAB	HUMAN eats FISH	HUMAN cuts skin SWIMMING
↓	↓	↓	↓
F. hepatica & *F. buska*	*P. westermani*	*C. sinensis* & *H. heterophyes*	Schisto-somes

How do schistosomes enter the body?
Via a split (schisto) in the body (soma). They enter via a break in the skin, not orally.

What causes "river blindness?"
Onchocerca volvulus:

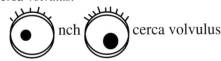

Everything goes BLACK (it's carried by the BLACKfly)

What is Paragonimus westermani*?*
The WESTERN MAN is the rugged Marlboro cigarette man, who gets LUNG disease, and ultimately cancer (the CRAB is the astrological sign of cancer). Hence, *P. westermani* is the LUNG fluke, which is carried by CRABS.

What are the ASH worms?

These three nematodes cause Leuffler's eosinophilia:

A S H

Ascaris:
- So big, it can block the gut
- Floats freely in the lumen

Strongyloides:
- *Strong* enough to live entirely in the soil without a host
- *Strong* enough to burrow through the skin, where it causes ground itch
- *Strong* enough to burrow through the gut wall and seed

Hookworms:
- The bloodsuckers
- *Hook* onto skin and penetrate
- Cause microcytic anemia by sucking blood from the gut

What is whipworm?
The sound of a whip is "TRICH TRICH," as in *Trichuris trichiura.*

I'll do a magic TRICK and swallow a football. This causes PROLAPSED RECTUM when the football finally comes out; *Trich trich* has a football-shaped ovum, and also causes prolapsed rectum.

How is Anisakis transmitted?
You get ani**SAKI**s by eating sushi (raw fish) with **SAKI**.

What are the major Jones criteria?

> **J** oint pain
> ♥ (carditis)
> **N** odules subcutaneously
> **E** rythema marginatum
> **S** ydenham's chorea

MICROBIOLOGY AND IMMUNOLOGY QUIZ

1. Which is incorrect regarding B cells?
    a. Upon exposure to an antigen, they express IgM first, then IgG
    b. They are deficient in men with Bruton's agammaglobulinemia
    c. They are produced by tissue surrounding the germinal centers
    d. B cell deficiency predisposes one to bacterial infections

2. Which is correctly matched concerning hypersensitivity?
    a. Type one involves complex deposition
    b. Type two is called delayed type
    c. Type three has an immediate onset
    d. Type four is T cell mediated

3. Which is correct?
    a. In a cell wall, the peptides bind to NAM
    b. Teichoic acid is more common in gram negative than positive
    c. Pili are more common in gram positive than negative
    d. Spores are more common in gram negative than positive

4. Which is incorrectly matched?
   a. Neisseria is a gram negative cocci
   b. Actinomyces is a gram positive anaerobic cocci
   c. *Corynebacterium diphtheria* is a gram positive aerobic rod
   d. *E. coli* is a gram negative rod

5. Group B streptococcus is most commonly associated with:
   a. the neonate
   b. the immunocompromised
   c. alcoholics
   d. IV drug abusers

6. Which is aerobic?
   a. Clostridium
   b. Bacillus
   c. Actinomyces
   d. Bacteroides

7. Which is gram negative?
   a. Clostridium
   b. Bacillus
   c. Actinomyces
   d. Bacteroides

For questions 8-12, match the following drugs with their correct attributes:
   a. Isoniazid
   b. Rifampin
   c. Pyrazinamide
   d. Ethambutol
   e. Tetracycline

8. Inhibits mycolic acid synthesis

9. Requires B6 supplement

10. Blocks tRNA

11. Colors contact lenses orange/red

12. Blocks RNA synthesis

13. Mycoplasma can be identified by all of the following except:
    a. "Fried egg" colonies
    b. Presence of cholesterol in membrane
    c. Positive cold agglutinin test
    d. Stains gram negative

14. Which is true regarding *Neisseria meningitidis*?
    a. It is oxidase negative.
    b. It is unencapsulated on CSF staining.
    c. It ferments both maltose and glucose.
    d. It is a gram negative rod.

For questions 15-18, match the following organisms with their correct attributes:
    a. *Campylobacter jejuni*
    b. *Staph aureus*
    c. Salmonella
    d. Shigella
    e. *Vibrio cholerae*
    f. *Clostridium perfringens*

15. Six members of a football team present with acute onset of nausea and emesis about three hours after a lunch cookout

16. Diarrhea caused by heat-resistant spores

17. The stool sample of a patient with diarrhea shows organisms that are motile but not C- or S-shaped

18. A patient experiences profuse watery diarrhea after eating sushi

19. A 43-year-old married man presents with a painless ulcer of his penis and multiple dark spots on his palms. He denies extramarital sex. He most likely has:
    a. *H. ducreyi*
    b. Bacterial endocarditis
    c. Lyme disease
    d. Syphilis

20. Several weeks later, the above patient develops painful knee and ankle joints and conjunctivitis. He is afebrile. The most logical diagnosis is:
    a. Previous coinfection with chlamydia
    b. Pseudogout
    c. Rheumatic fever
    d. Lyme disease

21. Which is incorrectly matched?
    a. Lyme disease: the migrating rash
    b. Coxsackie A (herpangina): rash of hands and feet only
    c. Rocky Mountain Spotted Fever: rash on trunk that progresses to extremities
    d. Measles: spots on buccal mucosa can be diagnostic

22. Which appears as a broad-based budding yeast?
    a. Coccidioidomycosis
    b. Blastomycosis
    c. Histoplasmosis
    d. Sporothrix

For questions 23-26, match the virus with its correct attribute:
    a. Herpes simplex
    b. EBV
    c. Hepatitis C
    d. CMV
    e. Poliovirus

23. Acquired by oral ingestion

24. Commonly responsible for retinitis

25. Yields a positive Tzanck smear

26. May cause leukoplakia

27. Which is true regarding a person with rabies:
    a. Tries to bite other people
    b. May have acquired it from a pet hamster or rabbit
    c. Is thirsty but unable to drink water
    d. Could have identified and thus avoided the rabid bats by their aberrant behavior

For questions 28-35, match the correct organism with each of the following descriptions:
    a. *Toxoplasma gondii*
    b. *Trypanosoma cruzi*
    c. *Taenia solium*
    d. *Naegleria fowleri*
    e. *Clonorchis sinensis* (fish tapeworm)
    f. *Paragonimus westermani*
    g. *Strongyloides*
    h. *Trichuris trichiura*
    i. *Onchocerca volvulus*
    j. *Taenia saginata*

28. Whipworm

29. A TORCH agent; bradyzoite stage in the brain

30. Causes B12 deficiency

31. Transmitted by the blackfly

32. Able to reproduce and survive entirely in the dirt

33. Enters through the nose of a swimmer and infects the brain

34. Transmitted in uncooked pork

35. A human eats an infected crab

APPENDIX I: ANSWERS TO CHAPTER QUIZZES

Gross Anatomy Quiz, page 19:

1. b	6. b	11. c	16. c	21. d
2. a	7. c	12. b	17. c	22. a
3. d	8. a	13. c	18. g	23. c
4. b	9. d	14. d	19. d	24. a
5. c	10. e	15. a	20. f	25. c

Microanatomy and Embryology Quiz, page 33:

1. c	4. b	7. d	10. c	13. d
2. d	5. c	8. a	11. b	
3. a	6. d	9. d	12. a	

Neuroscience Quiz, page 47:

1. d	5. c	9. k	13. a	17. c
2. b	6. d	10. i	14. d	18. b
3. a	7. a	11. l	15. f	
4. d	8. b	12. k	16. b	

Biochemistry Quiz, page 65:

1. c	6. a	11. a	16. a	21. a
2. c	7. c	12. d	17. d	
3. d	8. d	13. c	18. d	
4. b	9. a	14. d	19. a	
5. e	10. c	15. b	20. b	

Physiology Quiz, page 75:

1. a	4. d	7. b	10. b	13. b
2. d	5. c	8. b	11. a	14. a
3. c	6. c	9. d	12. a	

Behavioral Sciences Quiz, page 81:

1. b	2. b	3. c	4. a	5. c

Pathology Quiz, page 101:

1. d	7. b	13. d	19. g	25. a
2. c	8. d	14. b	20. b	26. b
3. b	9. b	15. c	21. c	27. c
4. a	10. a	16. a	22. a	28. d
5. c	11. c	17. i	23. a	
6. d	12. e	18. f	24. d	

Pharmacology Quiz, page 133:

1. c	9. a	17. b	25. c	33. b
2. b	10. b	18. c	26. d	34. b
3. a	11. a	19. c	27. d	35. c
4. a	12. c	20. b	28. a	36. d
5. d	13. c	21. a	29. c	37. a
6. b	14. b	22. b	30. a	38. b
7. c	15. d	23. a	31. a	39. d
8. d	16. a	24. b	32. d	

Microbiology and Immunology Quiz, page 161:

1. c	8. a	15. b	22. b	29. a
2. d	9. a	16. f	23. e	30. e
3. a	10. e	17. c	24. d	31. i
4. b	11. b	18. e	25. a	32. g
5. a	12. b	19. d	26. b	33. d
6. b	13. d	20. a	27. c	34. c
7. d	14. c	21. c	28. h	35. f

INDEX

B

C

D

F

G

H

I

JKL

M

N

O

PQ

S